VEGETABLE COOKBOOK FOR VEGANS

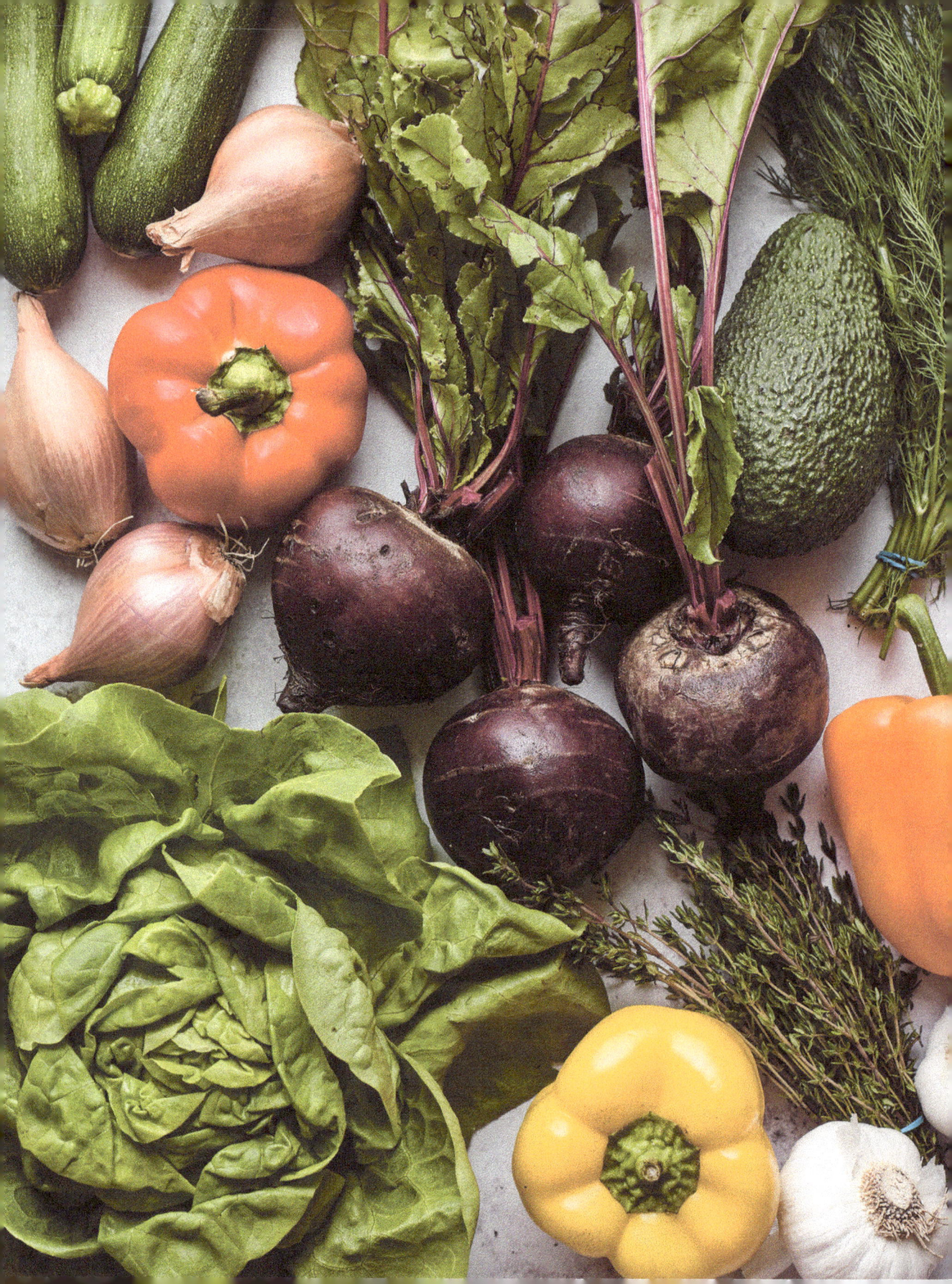

VEGETABLE COOKBOOK FOR VEGANS

100 Fresh and Easy Plant-Based Recipes

Larissa Olczak

Photography by Andrew Purcell

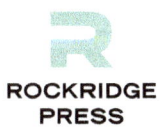

ROCKRIDGE PRESS

Copyright © 2021 by Rockridge Press, Emeryville, California

No part of this publication may be reproduced, stored in a retrieval system, or transmitted in any form or by any means, electronic, mechanical, photocopying, recording, scanning, or otherwise, except as permitted under Sections 107 or 108 of the 1976 United States Copyright Act, without the prior written permission of the Publisher. Requests to the Publisher for permission should be addressed to the Permissions Department, Rockridge Press, 6005 Shellmound Street, Suite 175, Emeryville, CA 94608.

Limit of Liability/Disclaimer of Warranty: The Publisher and the author make no representations or warranties with respect to the accuracy or completeness of the contents of this work and specifically disclaim all warranties, including without limitation warranties of fitness for a particular purpose. No warranty may be created or extended by sales or promotional materials. The advice and strategies contained herein may not be suitable for every situation. This work is sold with the understanding that the Publisher is not engaged in rendering medical, legal, or other professional advice or services. If professional assistance is required, the services of a competent professional person should be sought. Neither the Publisher nor the author shall be liable for damages arising herefrom. The fact that an individual, organization, or website is referred to in this work as a citation and/or potential source of further information does not mean that the author or the Publisher endorses the information the individual, organization, or website may provide or recommendations they/it may make. Further, readers should be aware that websites listed in this work may have changed or disappeared between when this work was written and when it is read.

For general information on our other products and services or to obtain technical support, please contact our Customer Care Department within the United States at (866) 744-2665, or outside the United States at (510) 253-0500.

Rockridge Press publishes its books in a variety of electronic and print formats. Some content that appears in print may not be available in electronic books, and vice versa.

TRADEMARKS: Rockridge Press and the Rockridge Press logo are trademarks or registered trademarks of Callisto Media Inc. and/or its affiliates, in the United States and other countries, and may not be used without written permission. All other trademarks are the property of their respective owners. Rockridge Press is not associated with any product or vendor mentioned in this book.

Interior and Cover Designer: Jill Lee
Art Producer: Meg Baggott
Editor: Gurvinder Singh Gandu
Production Editor: Rachel Taenzler
Production Manager: Michael Kay

Photography © 2021 Andrew Purcell. Food Styling by Carrie Purcell. Vegetable images, Shutterstock.

ISBN: Print 978-1-64876-449-3 | eBook 978-1-64876-450-9

R0

CONTENTS

INTRODUCTION *xi*

Part I: Vegetable Cooking Essentials *1*

The Joy of Vegetables *2*

Shopping for Flavor *2*

Vegetable Cooking Methods *5*

Tools of the Veggie Trade *6*

Part II: The Vegetables and Their Recipes *9*

Artichokes *10*

Simple Steamed Artichokes *11*

Roasted Baby Artichokes *13*

Arugula *14*

Arugula Salsa Verde *15*

Sautéed Arugula with Roasted Red Peppers *16*

Asparagus *17*

Shaved Asparagus and Pine Nut Salad *18*

Asparagus Soup with Peas *19*

Linguine with Asparagus *20*

Avocado *21*

Pineapple Avocado Salad *22*

Avocado Toast with Quick Pickled Red Onions *23*

Beets *24*

Coconut Curry Golden Beet Soup *25*

Beet Fries with Garlic Tahini *27*

Bok Choy *28*

Sautéed Bok Choy *29*

Roasted Baby Bok Choy with Spicy Maple Miso *30*

Broccoli 31

Cilantro-Lime Riced Broccoli 32

Steamed Broccoli with Peanut Sauce 33

Teriyaki Tofu and Roasted Broccoli 34

Broccolini 35

Broccolini Pasta Salad 36

Broccoli Rabe 37

Classic Sautéed Broccoli Rabe 38

Brussels Sprouts 39

Shredded Brussels Sprouts Salad 41

Turmeric Riced Brussels Sprouts 42

Cabbage 43

Braised Cabbage, Apples, and White Beans 44

Quick Sesame-Soy Red Cabbage Slaw 45

Carrots 46

Cardamom-Maple Roasted Baby Carrots 47

Roasted Carrot and Tahini Dressing 48

Salt and Vinegar Carrot Crisps 49

Cauliflower and Romanesco 50

Turmeric Cauliflower Steaks 51

Spiced Cauliflower, Chickpea, and Raisin Salad 52

Cauliflower Mac 'n' "Cheese" 53

Celery 54

Celery with Almond Butter and Pomegranate Arils 55

Celery Root 56

Garlicky Celery Root and Potato Soup 57

Chard 58

Maple Chard Salad 60

Chicories 61

Escarole and White Bean Soup 62

Corn 63

Corn Chowder 64

Fresh Corn and Cherry Dip 65

Cucumbers 66

Spicy Cucumber, Cashew, and Edamame Salad 67

Cucumber-Melon Salsa 68

Eggplant 69

Eggplant Bacon 70

Eggplant Parmesan 71

Japanese Eggplant with Thai Basil 72

Endive 73

Braised Endive 74

Fava Beans 75

Mashed Fava Bean Bruschetta 77

Marinated Fava Beans 78

Fennel 79

Roasted Fennel and Tomatoes over Pasta 80

Garlic 81

Roasted Garlic Bulbs 82

All-Purpose Garlic Marinade 83

Ginger 84

Homemade Candied Ginger 85

Green Beans 86

Blackened Green Beans 87

Green Beans and Potatoes 88

Herbs 89

Frozen Olive Oil and Rosemary Cubes 91

DIY Dried Herbs 92

Homemade Chimichurri 93

Jicama 94

Baked Jicama Fries with Homemade Chimichurri 95

Jicama-Mango Salsa 96

Kale, Collards, and Other Greens 97

Coconut Braised Kale 98

Crispy Kale Chips 99

Sautéed Mustard Greens 100

Gumbo Z'Herbes 101

Kohlrabi 102

Kohlrabi Noodles with Red Sauce and Kidney Beans 103

Leeks and Scallions 104

Roasted Leeks 105

Scallion Pancakes 106

Lettuce 107

Vermicelli Lettuce Wraps 109

Grilled Romaine Lettuce 110

Mushrooms 111

Balsamic Roasted Mushrooms 112

Mushroom Chips 113

Mushroom and Lentil Gravy 114

Portobello Burgers 115

Okra 116

Okra Curry 117

Onions and Shallots 118

Make-Ahead Caramelized Onions 119

Quick Pickled Red Onions 121

French Lentil and Shallot Soup 122

Parsnips 123

Thyme Roasted Parsnip Coins 124

Parsnip and Apple Soup 125

Peas and Peapods 126

Sautéed Green Peas with Dill 127

Snap Pea and Barley Salad with Shallot Dijon Vinaigrette 128

Peppers 129

Roasted Red Peppers 130

Fresh Bell Pepper and Herb Salad 131

Stuffed Pepper Soup 132

Potatoes 133

Olive Oil Purple Potato Salad 135

Paprika Baked Potato Chips 136

Scalloped Potatoes 137

Radishes 138

Tarragon Roasted Radishes 139

Radish Chips 140

Rhubarb 141

Rhubarb and Candied Ginger Jam 142

Rutabaga 143

Shaved Rutabaga and Peanut Salad 144

Spinach 145

Easy Wilted Spinach 146

Spinach and White Bean Stir-Fry 147

Sprouts and Microgreens *148*

Citrusy Microgreens *149*

Sweet Potatoes *150*

Sweet Potato and Chickpea Curry *151*

Sweet Potato Pizza Crust *153*

Sweet Potato Gnocchi *154*

Tomatillos *155*

Posole Verde *156*

Tomatoes *157*

Homemade Tomato Sauce *158*

Garden Tomato Soup *159*

Turnips *160*

Maple-Mustard Roasted Turnips *161*

Pureed Turnip and Garlic Dip *162*

Winter Squash *163*

Acorn Squash with Cranberry and Wild Rice Stuffing *164*

Spaghetti Squash with Kale and Chickpeas *165*

Pumpkin Pasta Carbonara *166*

Zucchini and Summer Squash *167*

Zucchini Pesto Pasta *169*

Zucchini Boats *170*

MEASUREMENT CONVERSIONS *173*

INDEX *174*

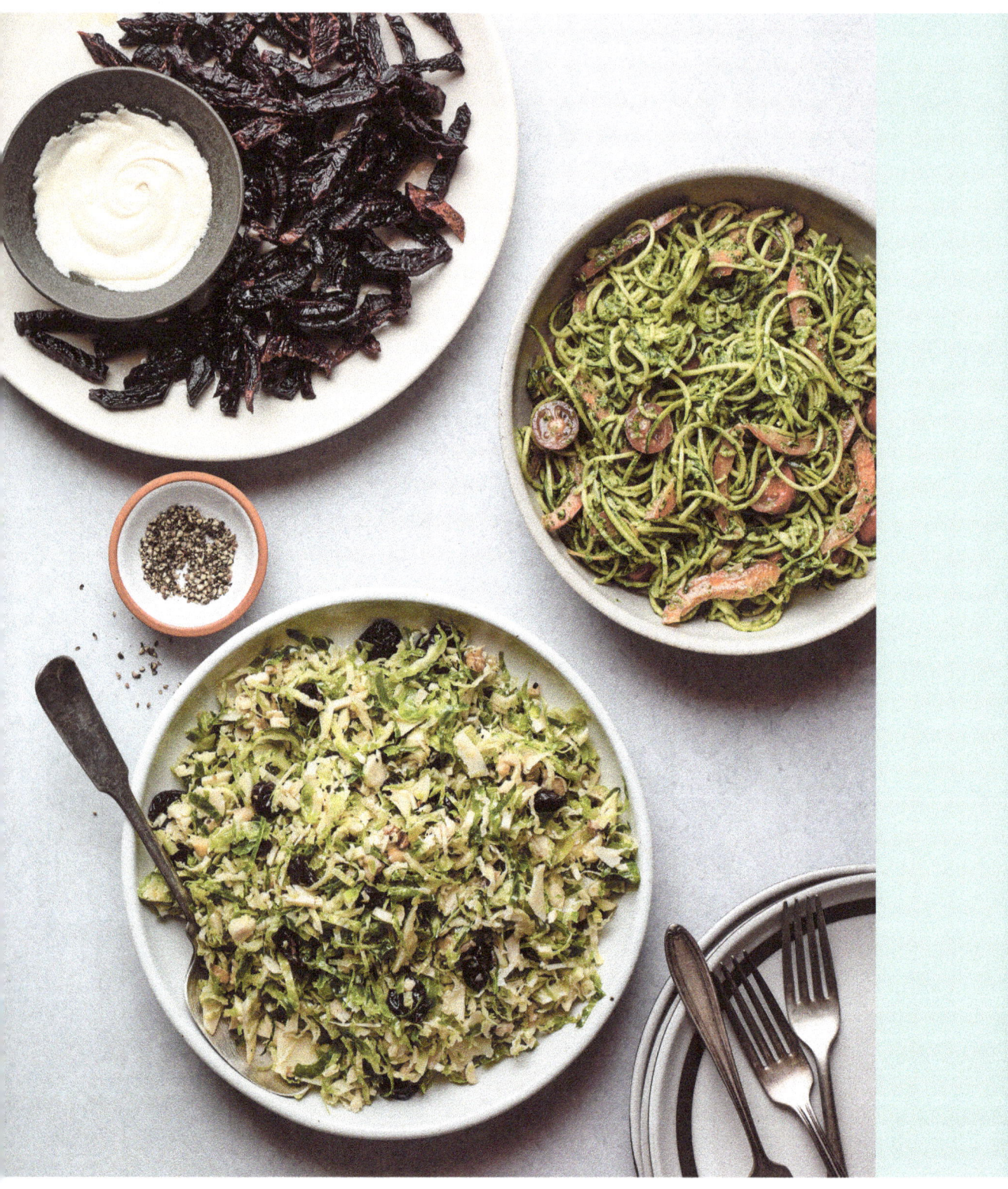

INTRODUCTION

There's no limit to the number of amazing plant-based recipes you can create. One of the many great things about vegetables is that they offer a vibrant range of tastes and textures, from sweet to savory and creamy to crunchy. To keep things interesting, each season provides us with different vegetables, so you can change things up throughout the year. Each vegetable offers a unique flavor profile and can be prepared in a variety of different ways—such as steamed, baked, roasted, sautéed, broiled, and even raw—and I'll show you which recipes work best with each vegetable. You can even put a new spin on traditionally animal-based recipes. With the right seasoning and kitchen appliances, you can make vegetables taste like cheese and even meat, creating the perfect plant-based substitute.

Often when people are trying to incorporate more vegetables into their lives, they feel overwhelmed and don't know where to start. This cookbook helps make that transition much simpler, with recipes made specifically to highlight the profile of each vegetable and easy tips on how to cook them. Did you ever imagine you'd be making a "cheese" sauce from cauliflower or a gluten-free pizza crust from sweet potatoes? I'll show you how. The good thing about veggies is that they're very easy to prepare, and these versatile recipes are perfect for both the home cook and the more experienced chef.

This cookbook is a celebratory A-to-Z using 50 different vegetables to create 100 recipes. You'll learn how to make delicious vegetable-based meals for both sides and mains. In this book, the vegetable will create the main flavor of the dish without any overpowering ingredients like butter or bacon. My intention is to showcase what vegetables have to offer and demonstrate how they can hold their own in recipes without animal-based ingredients.

You don't have to be vegan to use this cookbook—though you'll find it especially helpful if you are. But even if you're simply looking for new ways to eat vegetables, there's plenty of inspiration in these recipes.

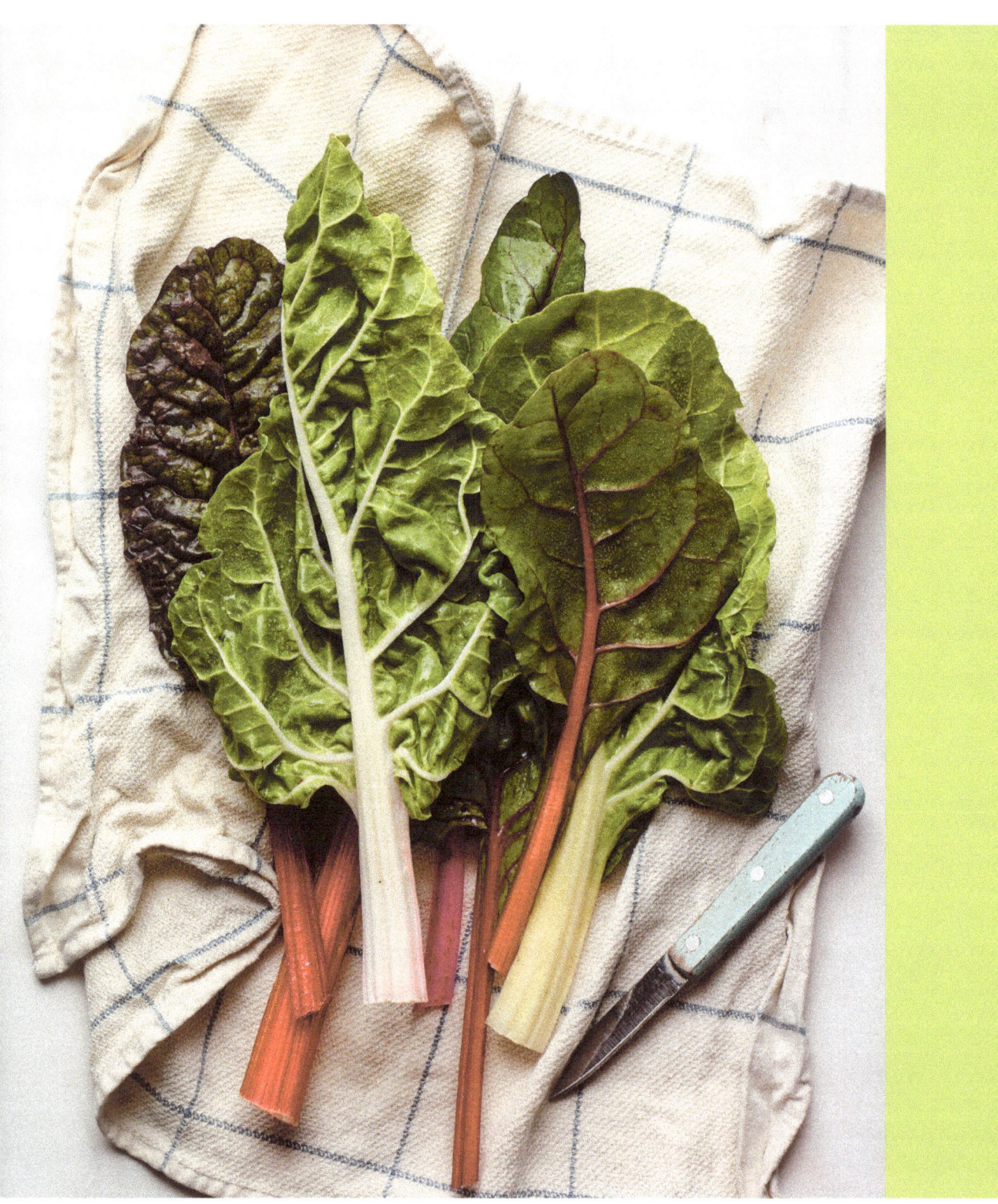

Chard, p. 58

PART I

VEGETABLE COOKING ESSENTIALS

The Joy of Vegetables

I can't stress enough the importance of the phrase "eat your veggies." There are so many to choose from, and this book will show you how to cook each one to completely satisfy you. As a Functional Nutritional Therapy Practitioner who supports a plant-based diet, I love sharing delicious vegan recipes to show people that you can be healthy without sacrificing flavor. There is a joy in eating vegetables because you're providing your body with the nutrients it needs to thrive. Plus, after eating a big plate of veggies, you're more likely to feel nourished instead of bloated or heavy. Back when you were a kid, eating your veggies might have seemed like a chore. But with the right cooking methods, kitchen appliances, and seasoning, they can be incredibly delicious.

Need more convincing? Well, consider the fact that vegetables are:

- A known factor in reducing the chances of developing chronic health conditions.

- An exciting culinary experience, with each vegetable offering its own unique flavor and texture.

- An amazing boost to your overall well-being by supporting a healthy, functioning gut; improving mood; decreasing inflammation; and more.

- A great way to support your community and local farmers.

Shopping for Flavor

It's important to know what to look for when shopping for quality produce. Make sure that the vegetables you're purchasing are bright in color, not limp, and don't have any spots or discoloration. Generally speaking, they should be slightly firm to the touch—you don't want anything that's soft or mushy.

Buying in Season

A good rule of thumb when shopping for produce is to shop seasonally. Each season offers an array of vegetables to enjoy. For example, during the colder months of fall and winter, you'll find more hearty root vegetables such as squashes, potatoes, and yams. During warmer months in spring and summer, you'll likely see lettuce, peas, artichokes, and asparagus at your local market. Eating seasonally ensures you are getting the vegetables at their peak, which is when they have the highest nutrient value.

Many vegetables don't have a discernible season, so you can enjoy them year-round, but the ones that are really better to buy in season are Brussels sprouts, bok choy, eggplants, and leeks.

Buying Local

Another perk of buying in season is that it allows you to support your local farmers and community. You can find seasonal produce at farmers' markets, through CSAs (community-supported agriculture), and usually at your neighborhood grocer. Even the big chains offer fresh seasonal produce, making it accessible for everyone.

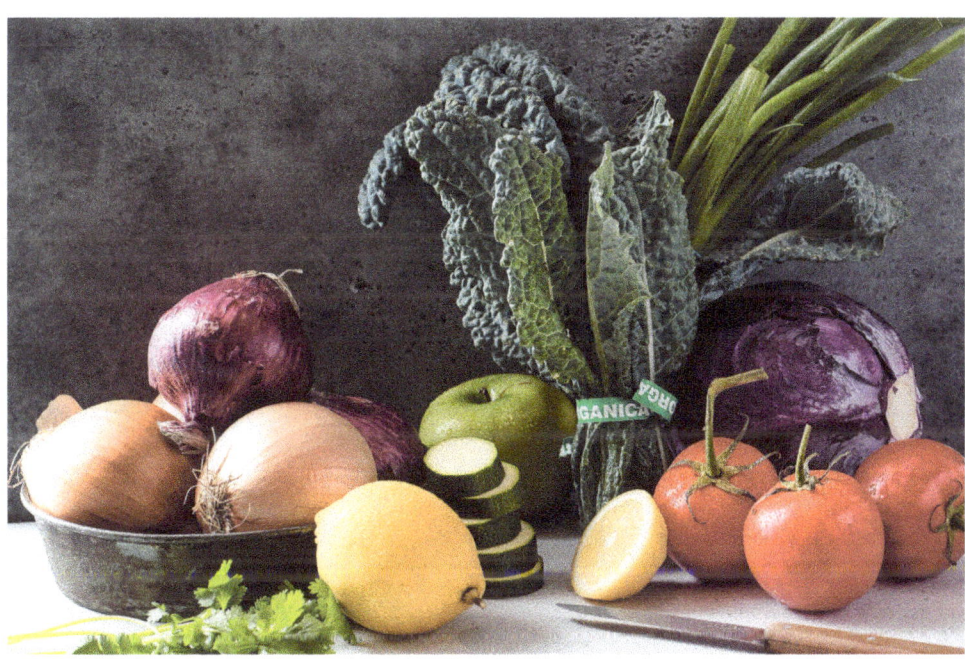

ADDING FLAVOR WITHOUT DAIRY OR EGGS

The good news is you don't *have* to use animal products like dairy, eggs, or bacon to bring out flavor in vegetable dishes. You can rely entirely on plant-based ingredients to make your meals taste amazing. Here are some secrets to doing that:

Vegetable broth/bouillon: This is an easy replacement in dishes that call for chicken broth. Vegetable broth gives that umami flavor to vegan dishes and can work great in soups, pastas, and even sauces.

Liquid smoke: This incorporates the same smoky/meaty flavor without the actual meat. It tastes amazing in dishes that have tofu, tempeh, or another vegan protein.

Nutritional yeast: This allows you to create that cheesy flavor in your dishes. Add a dash of turmeric to give it a yellow color so that it looks and tastes like real cheese. Blend with firm tofu to create a ricotta equivalent.

Unsweetened plant-based milk: This is the perfect replacement for milk. It tastes just like milk and also has a similar consistency. Opt for cashew or flaxseed milk for a higher fat content.

Coconut aminos/soy sauce: Adding these to your dishes, specifically stir-fries, is another great way to add in a savory umami flavor otherwise derived from meat.

Black salt: Black salt has a high sulfuric content, giving it the smell and flavor of eggs. Use in dishes that typically call for eggs—even with soft tofu to create vegan scrambled eggs.

Vegan butter: Just because you're vegan doesn't mean you have to give up butter entirely. The plant-based variety can be used in any recipes that traditionally call for regular butter.

Vegetable Cooking Methods

Not all veggies are created equal, and many of them require different cooking methods. Below are some of the most common vegetable cooking methods and the veggies they work best for.

ROASTING: When food reaches high heat, it browns and caramelizes. Roasting veggies can turn something hard and otherwise bland into something soft and full of mouthwatering flavor. Some great veggies to roast are cauliflower, potatoes, carrots, yams, broccoli, Brussels sprouts, squash, asparagus, and onions.

GRILLING: When you grill veggies, the smoke naturally provides a delicious flavor. You won't even need marinades or sauces, because the flavor will come from the vegetable itself. Some vegetables that are great for the grill are portobello mushrooms, zucchini, asparagus, onions, and bell peppers.

SAUTÉING: This is a common method for preparing vegetables and also one of the best ways to preserve the nutrients. You can chop the vegetables into smaller pieces and sauté on low heat (exposing your veggies to high heat can diminish the nutrient profile). It's best to sauté quick-cooking veggies, such as onions, broccoli, bell peppers, mushrooms, onions, celery, and green beans.

STIR-FRYING: Stir-frying is traditionally done in a wok, and it uses a short cooking time with high heat and oil. Common vegetables used for stir-fries are carrots, peas, onions, and broccoli.

BRAISING: To braise vegetables, you start off by sautéing them at a high temperature, then cover and cook them with liquid at a low temperature for a longer period. This will give you a delicious, soft, and saucy vegetable dish. Braising is great for potatoes, yams, and carrots.

STEAMING: Steaming is a great way to cook leafy greens and cruciferous vegetables like broccoli and cauliflower. Lightly steaming veggies also helps preserve the nutrients. Add a little bit of salt and lemon to create a delicious flavor.

Tools of the Veggie Trade

When cooking vegetables, it's important to be equipped with the proper kitchen tools. Here's what you should have on hand:

MANDOLINE: Using a mandoline helps create thin, even slices of veggies such as potatoes, bell peppers, or carrots.

GRILL BASKET: You can evenly grill your sliced or whole veggies by putting a grill basket on top of your grill.

SPIRALIZER: Make delicious noodle-like strands from veggies like zucchini to re-create spaghetti. You can also use a spiralizer on things like carrots to put on salads.

STEAMER: A must-have in the kitchen, a steamer allows you to easily steam many veggies at once.

WOK: A wok is necessary for a stir-fry. It gets hot quickly and allows the food to cook over high heat for short periods.

STAINLESS-STEEL PAN: This is a great pan for sautéing veggies and can be used over low, medium, and high heat.

CAST-IRON SKILLET: You can use this skillet to sauté, braise, and even roast vegetables.

HIGH-SPEED BLENDER: A blender is a must-have to create sauces and soups.

FOOD PROCESSOR: A food processor is a handy tool for making various dips and sauces.

SHEET PAN: This pan is necessary for roasting veggies and creating quick sheet pan dinners.

RICE COOKER: Many veggie meals are accompanied by rice, so having a rice cooker is an easy way to make perfect rice every time.

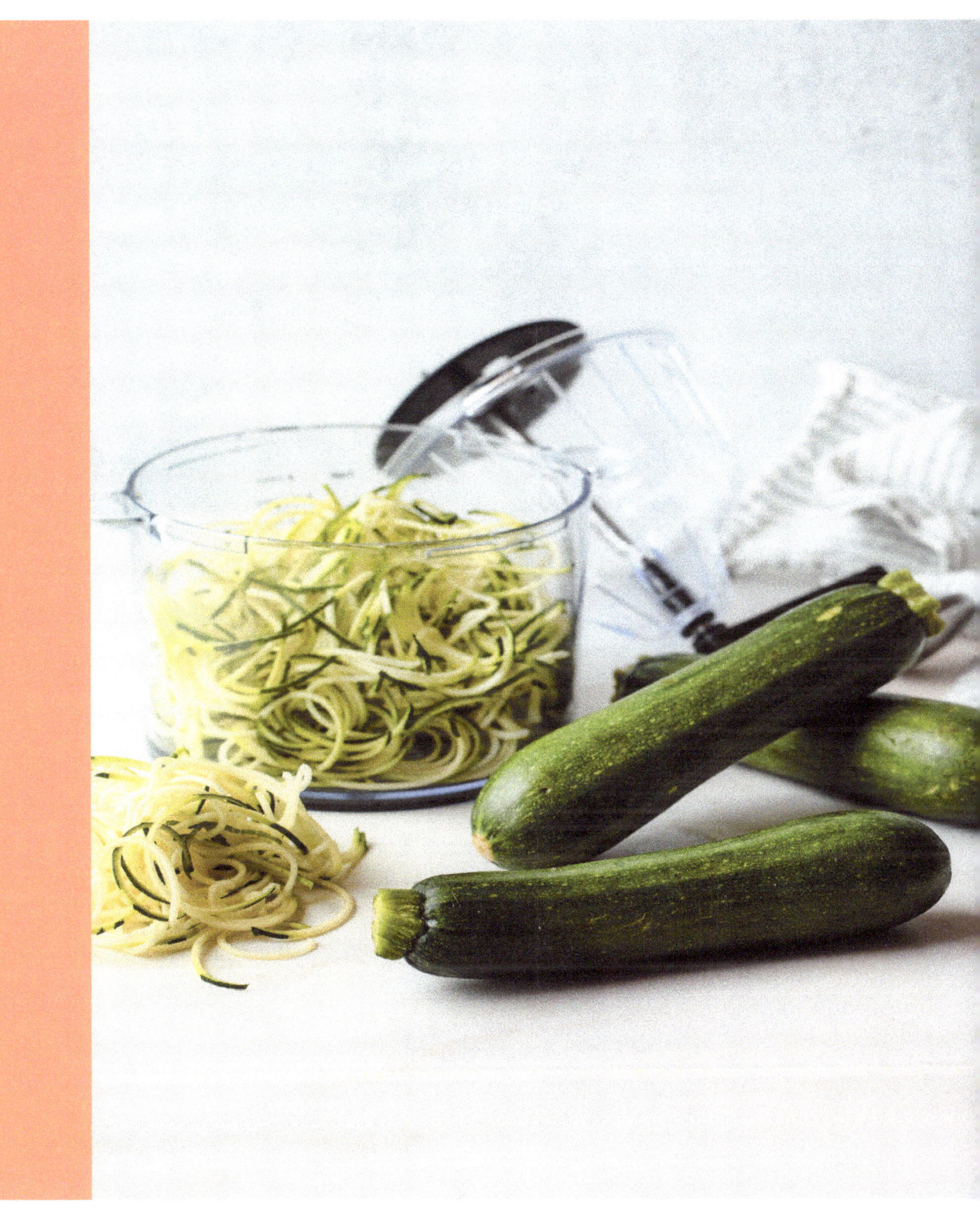

Zucchini and Summer Squash, p. 167

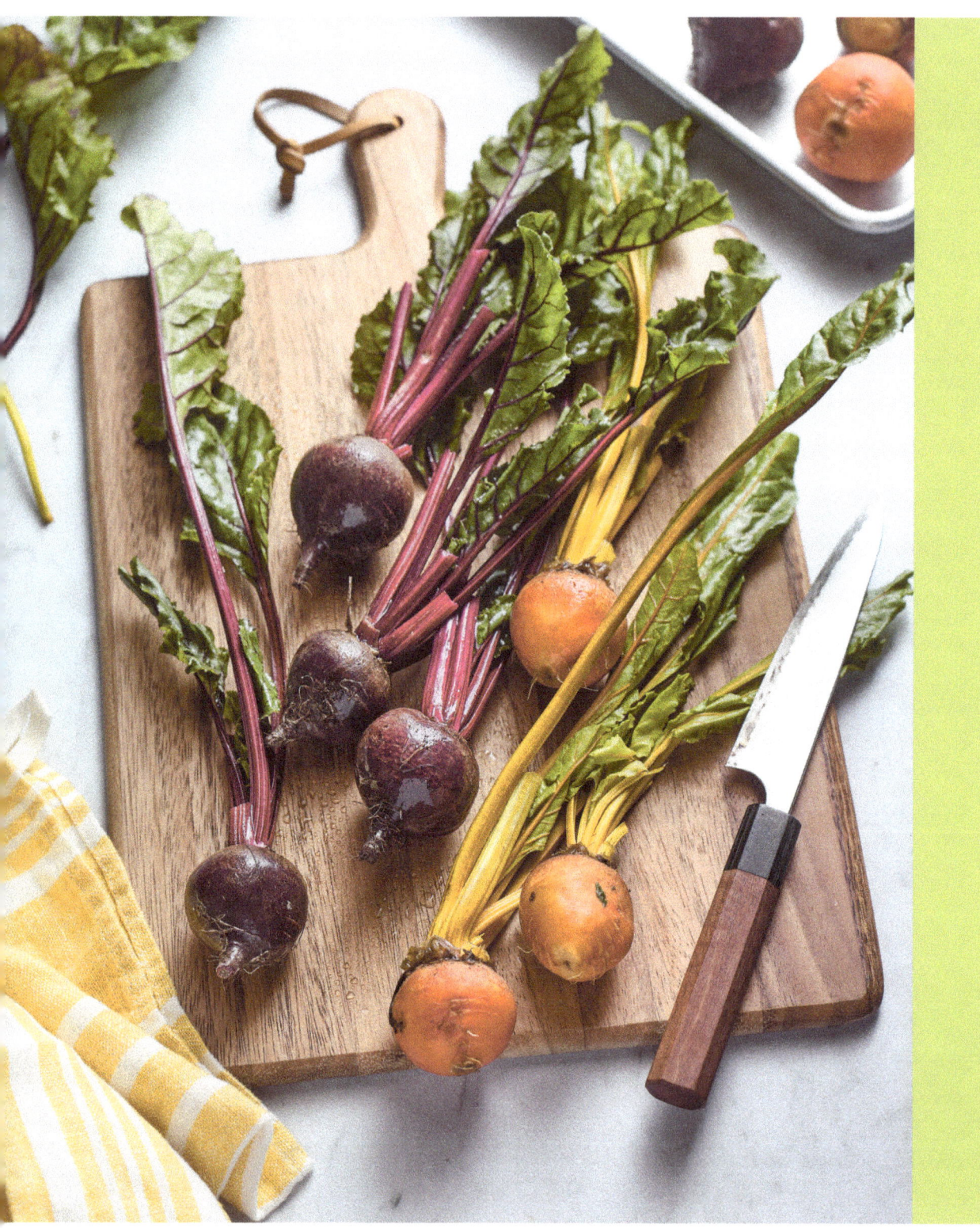

Beets, p. 24

PART II

THE VEGETABLES AND THEIR RECIPES

Artichokes

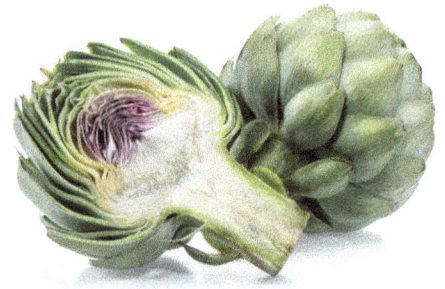

Season: Spring

Flavor profile: Artichokes are a type of thistle with beautiful green, edible outer leaves that surround a tender "heart." The heart sits on top of the stem and has a fuzzy, inedible center called a "choke." They have a rich flavor that's earthy and slightly sweet, and the heart is considered the most flavorful and meaty part.

Pairs with: Lemon, fresh herbs, and garlic.

Varieties: Globe (most popular, also known as round), baby (no fuzzy chokes!), and purple (several varieties).

Preparation: To prepare artichokes for cooking, have a serrated or sharp knife, fresh lemon wedges, and kitchen scissors handy. Once the artichokes are cooked, you can eat them by removing the leaves and using your teeth to scrape away the tender flesh. Discard the tough leaves after eating the flesh, but eat the heart whole.

Favorite cooking methods: Roasted, steamed, and braised.

Nutritional info: Artichokes are high in vitamin C, magnesium, and inulin, a dietary fiber that acts as a prebiotic and can feed healthy gut bacteria.

Selection: Look for artichokes that are heavy and have tight leaves that have not opened. To test an artichoke's freshness, give it a firm squeeze. If it squeaks, you have a fresh one.

Storage: Store raw artichokes in a plastic bag, poked with a few holes, in the refrigerator for 5 to 7 days. Cooked artichokes are best eaten right away but can last in an airtight container in the refrigerator for a few days.

Simple Steamed Artichokes

Serves 4 | Prep time: 10 minutes | Cook time: 25 minutes

These leafy, mild-flavored veggies taste amazing steamed. Steaming brings out the nutty flavor and light buttery sweetness.

4 fresh artichokes

1 lemon, quartered

1. Using a sharp or serrated knife, cut off about ½ inch from both the top and stem of each artichoke. Remove the tough outer leaves toward the bottom. Use kitchen scissors to snip the pointy tops of the other leaves. Rub the cut surfaces with a slice of lemon to prevent browning.

2. Fill a large pot with a few of inches of water and squeeze some lemon juice into it. Place a vegetable steamer basket into the pot and put the artichokes in the basket. If you don't have a basket, put the artichokes directly into the pot, stem-side up. Bring to a boil over high heat. Lower the heat to medium-low, cover, and simmer for 25 to 35 minutes. The artichokes are finished cooking when the heart is fork-tender and you can easily peel off the leaves.

3. Enjoy a freshly steamed artichoke by dipping a leaf into a sauce of your choice and using your teeth to scrape away the tender flesh. The heart and stem are also edible, but the fuzzy choke should be discarded.

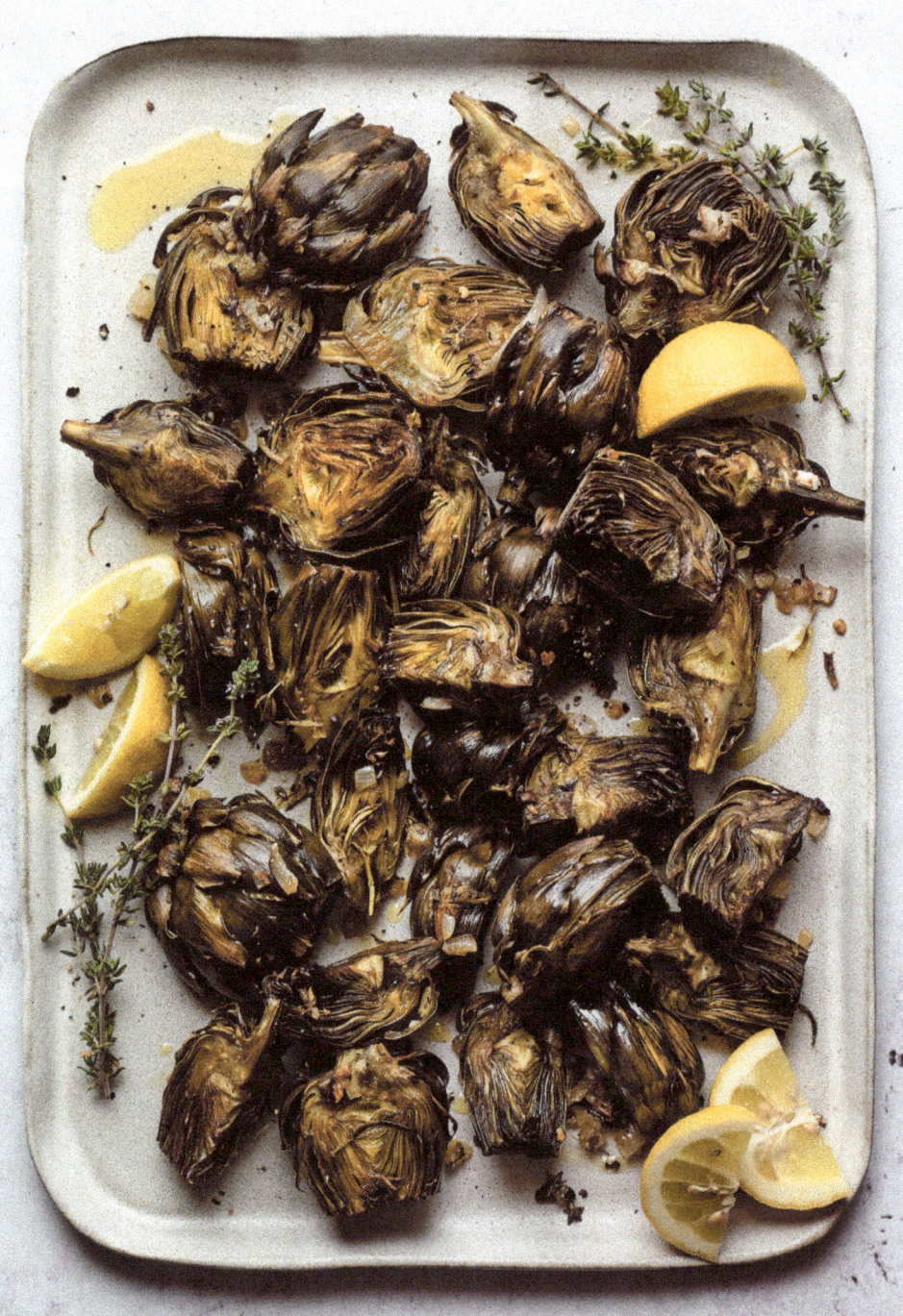

Roasted Baby Artichokes

Serves 4 | Prep time: 10 minutes | Cook time: 25 minutes

Compared to their larger counterparts, baby artichokes are much more tender and easier to cook. This recipe pairs them with lemon, herbs, and chili flakes and will change how you look at these petite vegetables.

8 baby artichokes

3 tablespoons extra-virgin olive oil

Zest and juice of ½ lemon

1 small shallot, minced

½ teaspoon fresh thyme leaves

½ teaspoon fresh rosemary

¼ teaspoon dried chili flakes

Himalayan salt

Freshly ground black pepper

1. Preheat the oven to 400°F.
2. Trim the stems of the artichokes and remove the tough outer leaves. Cut ½ inch off the top of each artichoke. Cut them in half or quarters depending on size.
3. Place the artichokes on a baking sheet. Drizzle with the olive oil, and sprinkle with the lemon zest, lemon juice, shallot, thyme, rosemary, and chili flakes. Season with salt and pepper. Toss well to coat evenly.
4. Bake, stirring halfway through, for about 25 minutes, or until tender.
5. Remove from the oven and season with additional salt.

Arugula

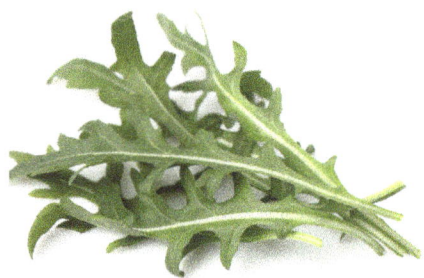

Season: Spring and Fall

Flavor profile: Arugula, also known as rocket, is a leafy green vegetable with a slightly spicy, peppery taste. It has hints of nuts and mustard and can be used both as a salad green and as an herb.

Pairs with: Olive oil, balsamic vinegar, lemon, almonds, pine nuts, sunflower seeds, pears, apples, oranges, and bell peppers.

Varieties: Common arugula (mostly found in the United States) and wild arugula (mostly found in Europe).

Preparation: Remove any wilted or yellow leaves. Wash arugula under cold water and pat dry with a clean towel before cooking.

Favorite cooking methods: Raw in salads and condiments, and sautéed.

Nutritional info: Arugula is an excellent source of vitamin K, a fat-soluble nutrient that's necessary for blood clotting. It also contains vitamin C, calcium, iron, and potassium.

Selection: Choose fresh arugula that has bright green leaves without yellow edges, wilting, or holes. Baby arugula has a milder and less bitter taste than bigger leaves that are left on the stem longer.

Storage: Wash and dry arugula before placing it between paper towels. Store in a plastic bag or airtight container in the refrigerator. Depending on how fresh it was when you got it, arugula can last for up to 10 days.

Arugula Salsa Verde

Makes 2 cups | Prep time: 15 minutes | Cook time: 10 minutes

In Italian tradition, salsa verde ("green sauce") is made with fresh parsley, garlic, onion, capers, and anchovies, while Mexican salsa verde features tomatillos, garlic, onion, cilantro, lime, and hot peppers. This recipe combines flavors from both types, resulting in something quite new. Although it may seem like a traditional Mexican salsa verde, it gets a peppery kick from one of the most loved greens in Italian cuisine—arugula.

- 1 pound tomatillos, husked and rinsed
- 3 cups loosely packed arugula, rinsed and dried
- 1 jalapeño, seeded and finely chopped
- ½ cup diced red onion
- 2 garlic cloves, minced, plus more as needed
- ¼ cup chopped fresh cilantro, plus more as needed
- Juice of 1 lime, plus more as needed
- ½ teaspoon salt, plus more as needed

1. Turn the broiler to high. Line a baking sheet with aluminum foil or parchment paper.
2. Place the tomatillos on the prepared baking sheet and broil for 5 to 7 minutes, or until their skins are lightly blackened and have black and brown marks.
3. Transfer the tomatillos and their juices to a food processor or blender. Add the arugula, jalapeño, onion, garlic, cilantro, lime juice, and salt. Pulse for 30 to 60 seconds, or until the salsa is finely chopped. Taste and add more salt, lime, garlic, or cilantro as desired.
4. Transfer to an airtight container and store in the refrigerator for up to 2 weeks. It will thicken the longer it is stored.

Notes: For a milder salsa, use half of the jalapeño or omit it altogether. For more spice, add another jalapeño or more arugula. Serve with tortilla chips, on top of tacos or burritos, or mixed into guacamole.

Sautéed Arugula with Roasted Red Peppers

Serves 4 | Prep time: 5 minutes | Cook time: 10 minutes

Sweet bell peppers complement spicy arugula in this easy side dish, and making the roasted red peppers in advance saves tons of time. Enjoy it alongside pasta, serve it on top of toasted bread, or bulk it up with white beans for a main dish. However you enjoy this recipe, be sure to add a drizzle of balsamic vinegar for a burst of flavor before serving.

- 1 tablespoon extra-virgin olive oil
- 3 garlic cloves, minced
- 6 cups loosely packed arugula, rinsed and dried
- 1 cup Roasted Red Peppers (page 130)
- Salt
- Freshly ground black pepper
- Balsamic vinegar, for serving

1. In a large skillet over medium heat, warm the olive oil. Add the garlic and cook for 1 to 2 minutes, or until fragrant.
2. Add the arugula and cook, stirring occasionally, for another 2 to 3 minutes, or until the arugula begins to wilt.
3. Add the red peppers and cook, stirring, for another 2 to 3 minutes.
4. Season with salt and pepper and drizzle with balsamic vinegar just before serving.

Notes: Arugula cooks down quickly, so use more if you have a lot on hand. Possible additions include red pepper flakes, mushrooms, fresh parsley, and onion.

Asparagus

Season: Spring

Flavor profile: Asparagus is a spear-like vegetable with pointy, scaly tips. It is a member of the lily family and comes in a variety of colors. Fresh asparagus has a mild, earthy taste but can taste bitter or sour when overcooked. Its mellow flavor allows it to soak up other flavors and seasonings particularly well.

Pairs with: Garlic, lemon, tarragon, mint, dill, soy, sesame, and balsamic vinegar.

Varieties: Green (garden), purple, and white.

Preparation: Rinse asparagus under water and snap off or trim the bottom of the spears with a knife to remove any woody or white/discolored parts.

Favorite cooking methods: Shaved, steamed, sautéed, and roasted.

Nutritional info: Asparagus contains fiber, potassium, and vitamins A, C, E, and K. It is particularly high in folate, which is an important nutrient for expecting moms due to its role in promoting healthy fetal development.

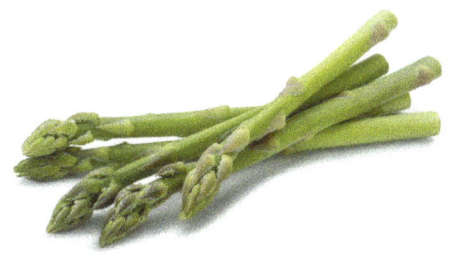

Selection: Look for asparagus that has firm stalks with tightly closed tips and few woody ends. Thin asparagus spears taste especially good in roasted and sautéed dishes; thicker stalks work well for shaved preparations and pastas, risottos, and soups.

Storage: Fill a glass jar with a couple of inches of water and store the asparagus spears upright in the refrigerator for up to 4 days. Or wrap the ends with a damp paper towel and place the bunch in a perforated plastic bag.

Shaved Asparagus and Pine Nut Salad

Serves 4 | Prep time: 15 minutes | Cook time: 5 minutes

Raw asparagus is a true springtime treat. It's sweet, mild, and downright delicious. Shaved asparagus is also a beautiful style of presentation. This simple side is easy enough for a weeknight meal and elegant enough to impress guests at a spring-inspired dinner. Before you get started, have a swivel peeler or sharp paring knife on hand to make the signature "ribbons" for this salad.

FOR THE SALAD

- 1 pound asparagus, trimmed (about 1 bunch)
- ¼ cup pine nuts

FOR THE DRESSING

- 2 tablespoons extra-virgin olive oil
- 1 teaspoon Dijon mustard
- 1 tablespoon freshly squeezed lemon juice
- Salt
- Freshly ground black pepper

TO MAKE THE SALAD

1. Lay the asparagus flat on a cutting board. Hold a spear down with one hand while you use your other hand to make long shavings with a vegetable peeler (or knife). There will be some uneven pieces, especially as you get toward the end of the stalk, but don't throw them out. You can cut them into smaller pieces and add them to the salad. Place the shaved asparagus in a bowl.

2. In a skillet over medium heat, toast the pine nuts, stirring frequently, for 2 to 3 minutes, or until fragrant. Add the pine nuts to the asparagus.

TO MAKE THE DRESSING

3. In a small bowl, whisk together the olive oil, mustard, and lemon juice. Season with salt and pepper to taste.

4. Add the dressing to the salad and toss to combine. Taste and season with more salt and pepper if desired.

Notes: Possible additions include chopped fresh parsley or mint. You can also use almonds instead of pine nuts. This tastes best immediately after preparation but can be stored in an airtight container in the refrigerator for up to 3 days.

Asparagus Soup with Peas

Serves 4 | Prep time: 10 minutes | Cook time: 30 minutes

This vibrant soup is like spring in a bowl. I've added the peas after blending to give texture. While this soup is tasty enough on its own, a thick piece of crunchy bread for dipping makes it even better.

1 tablespoon extra-virgin olive oil

1 sweet onion, diced

2 garlic cloves, minced

Salt

Freshly ground black pepper

1 pound asparagus, trimmed and cut into 1-inch pieces (about 1 bunch)

4 cups vegetable broth

1 cup frozen or fresh peas

2 tablespoons chopped fresh dill, plus more for serving

1. In a large pot over medium heat, warm the olive oil. Add the onion and garlic and sauté for 3 to 4 minutes, or until soft. Season with salt and pepper.

2. Add the asparagus and broth and stir to combine. Raise the heat to high, cover, and bring to a boil. Lower the heat to medium-low and cook for 20 to 25 minutes, or until the asparagus is fork-tender. Add more salt and pepper as desired.

3. Turn off the heat and, using an immersion blender, puree the soup. Add the peas and dill, stir to combine, and turn the heat back on to medium. Cook for 3 to 5 minutes, or until the soup is warmed through and the peas are tender. Serve with more dill.

Notes: You can also use a regular blender for this recipe. To do this safely, fill the blender halfway and puree the soup in batches. Leave a corner of the lid cracked or remove the top of the blender and cover it with a folded dish towel to let steam escape as you blend. Be careful not to get burned by the steam. Transfer the soup back to the pot and continue with the rest of the recipe.

Linguine with Asparagus

Serves 2 | Prep time: 20 minutes | Cook time: 45 minutes

Traditionally, it's the dairy in linguine dishes that gives them that creamy flavor. Fortunately, you can easily create that same flavor using vegan ingredients. The cauliflower and cashew sauce pairs perfectly with the linguine noodles, lemon, and asparagus.

1 bunch asparagus, trimmed ½ inch

1½ tablespoons extra-virgin olive oil, divided

1½ teaspoons Himalayan salt, divided

¾ teaspoon freshly ground black pepper, divided

2 medium lemons, thinly sliced

1 cup cashews

1 box gluten-free linguine noodles

1 large yellow onion, chopped

3 large garlic cloves, minced

½ cup vegetable broth

2 cups chopped cauliflower

Juice of ½ lemon

4 tablespoons nutritional yeast

½ lemon, for serving

1. Preheat the oven to 400°F.
2. Spread out the asparagus on a baking sheet and toss with ½ tablespoon of olive oil, ½ teaspoon of salt, and ½ teaspoon of pepper. Top with several thin slices of lemon and bake for 20 minutes. Once the asparagus has finished cooking, remove it from the oven and roughly chop it into thirds.
3. Bring a pot of water to a boil and boil the cashews for 15 minutes. Drain and set aside.
4. While the cashews are boiling, cook the pasta according to the package instructions.
5. In a large skillet over medium heat, warm the remaining 1 tablespoon of olive oil. Add the onion and garlic and sauté for 7 minutes, or until brown.
6. Add the broth and cauliflower to the skillet. Reduce the heat to low, cover, and cook for 10 minutes, or until the cauliflower is fork-tender.
7. Transfer the cauliflower mixture to a high-speed blender or food processor. Add the boiled cashews, the lemon juice, the remaining 1 teaspoon of salt, the remaining ¼ teaspoon of pepper, and the nutritional yeast and blend until smooth. Taste and adjust the seasoning if desired.
8. In a medium bowl, combine the sauce, asparagus, and noodles. Stir until coated evenly. Squeeze half a lemon over the top just before serving.

Avocado

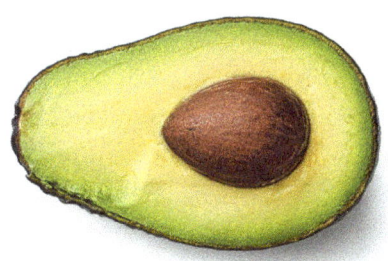

Season: Spring and Summer

Flavor profile: Avocados have creamy, bright green flesh with a brown pit and black or green skin. Botanically, they're considered a fruit, but they're typically eaten as a vegetable. Avocados have a rich, earthy, and slightly sweet flavor, and they contribute a buttery texture to dips, sauces, and smoothies.

Pairs with: Lime and lemon juice, garlic, onions, spicy peppers, beans, and chocolate.

Varieties: Hass (sourced from Mexico and California), Fuerte (green skin), and Florida (also known as Dominican, with green skin, larger pits, and lower fat content), as well as several other types that range from pear-shaped to oval.

Preparation: Cut an avocado in half lengthwise from stem to end, rotating it with one hand while keeping your knife steady with the other. Twist the avocado open with your hands, tap the knife firmly into the pit, and twist the knife to dislodge it. Scoop the flesh out with a spoon.

Favorite cooking methods: Mashed into guacamole, served on toast, and in salads.

Nutritional info: Avocados are known for being high in heart-healthy monounsaturated fats, but they are also a source of potassium and magnesium that help maintain healthy blood pressure.

Selection: To figure out whether an avocado is ripe, gently press your thumb into the skin. It should feel soft but not mushy. The skin of Hass avocados gets darker as they ripen, but this does not happen with most other varieties.

Storage: Unripe avocados should be stored on the countertop for up to 6 days, until ripe, then transferred to the refrigerator for up to 4 days. To store half of an avocado for later use, brush the flesh with lemon juice or olive oil to prevent browning, tightly wrap with plastic wrap, and place in the refrigerator.

Pineapple Avocado Salad

Serves 4 | Prep time: 15 minutes

Creamy avocados complement pineapple and serrano peppers in this warm-weather dish. Even though it's made with simple ingredients, the sweet, spicy, and cooling tastes, plus a touch of fresh dill, provide a variety of interesting flavors. You can serve it as a side to a summer cookout, eat it with tortilla chips, or add it to tacos and burrito bowls. Add some black beans to make it a complete meal.

FOR THE SALAD

- 2 ripe avocados, halved lengthwise, pits removed
- 3 cups diced pineapple
- 1 cup diced red onion
- 1 small serrano pepper, seeded and finely chopped
- 3 tablespoons chopped fresh dill

FOR THE DRESSING

- Juice of 2 limes
- 2 teaspoons maple syrup
- Salt

TO MAKE THE SALAD

1. Cut the avocado flesh into cubes and use a spoon to scoop it into a bowl. Add the pineapple, onion, serrano pepper, and dill and stir to combine.

TO MAKE THE DRESSING

2. In a small bowl, whisk together the lime juice and maple syrup.

3. Pour the dressing over the salad and mix until combined. Season with salt.

Notes: Use a jalapeño instead of a serrano pepper for less heat, or omit the pepper entirely. You can also substitute fresh cilantro in place of the dill.

Avocado Toast with Quick Pickled Red Onions

Serves 4 | Prep time: 5 minutes

When my husband and I visited Australia for our honeymoon, we fell in love with their take on avocado toast. Most restaurants served it on sourdough bread with pickled red onions, and sometimes they added sweet corn, crumbled feta, or a spice blend called dukkah, made with crushed nuts and seeds. Aussie-inspired avocado toast is now one of my favorite dishes to make for "brekkie." It tastes especially delicious alongside a cappuccino dusted with shaved chocolate, another Australian specialty.

4 large slices sourdough bread

2 avocados, halved lengthwise, pits removed

8 tablespoons Quick Pickled Red Onions (page 121)

4 tablespoons hemp seeds

1. Toast the sourdough bread in a toaster or under the broiler.
2. Scoop the flesh out of the avocados and, using a fork, mash it on top of each slice of toast. Divide the red onions and hemp seeds equally over the toasts. Enjoy!

Notes: If you can find dukkah at the store, add a sprinkle to the toast or use it instead of the hemp seeds. It is so delicious! You can also add corn, chopped cherry tomatoes, and/or a poached egg, and substitute rye or multigrain toast for the sourdough.

Beets

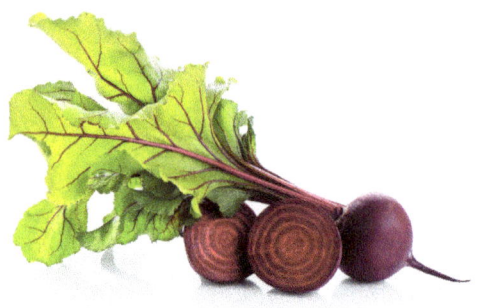

Season: Summer, Fall, and Winter

Flavor profile: Beets are a hearty root vegetable known for their earthy, yet slightly sweet, flavor. Raw beets have a more pronounced earthiness, while cooked beets taste sweeter. Beet greens are also edible and taste similar to other dark, leafy greens.

Pairs with: Savory herbs, walnuts, almonds, pistachios, pecans, and chocolate.

Varieties: Red (most popular), Chioggia (red-and-white-striped flesh), golden, and white.

Preparation: Trim beets with a sharp knife and peel or scrub with a vegetable brush. Red beets can stain your hands, but it will come off with soap and water. To avoid stains, wear gloves when handling.

Favorite cooking methods: Roasted whole or as fries, pureed into soup, and eaten raw and grated into slaws and salads.

Nutritional info: Beets are rich in fiber, folate, iron, and vitamin C. They also contain nitrates, which are beneficial compounds that may help reduce blood pressure and improve oxygen flow in the body.

Selection: Look for beets that are firm to the touch and do not have any dark bruises or blemishes. If their greens are intact, they should be healthy with strong stems and not wilted.

Storage: Beets can last for up to 4 weeks in a cool, dry place, such as a crisper drawer in the refrigerator. If you purchase beets with their greens, cut them off and use them within a few days.

Coconut Curry Golden Beet Soup

Serves 4 | Prep time: 10 minutes | Cook time: 40 minutes

Thanks to warm spices and velvety coconut milk, this deep yellow soup is the definition of comforting. Enjoy a bowl while you snuggle under a blanket to make it even better. Golden beets are considered by many to be slightly sweeter than their red counterparts, and a combination of curry powder, cumin, ginger, and cinnamon amplifies their sweetness. Add some paprika and some roasted chickpeas on top before serving.

1 tablespoon extra-virgin olive oil

1 sweet onion, diced

2 teaspoons curry powder

1 teaspoon ground cumin

½ teaspoon ground ginger

¼ teaspoon ground cinnamon

Salt

3 medium golden beets, scrubbed, trimmed, and chopped

4 cups vegetable broth

1 (13.5-ounce) can full-fat coconut milk

1. In a large pot or Dutch oven over medium heat, warm the olive oil. Add the onion and cook for 3 to 5 minutes, or until tender.
2. Sprinkle in the curry powder, cumin, ginger, and cinnamon, and cook, stirring frequently, for another 2 minutes, or until fragrant. Season with salt.
3. Add the golden beets and broth, raise the heat to high, and bring to a boil. Cover, lower the heat to medium-low, and cook for about 30 minutes, or until the beets are fork-tender.
4. Add the coconut milk and stir well. Turn off the heat. Using an immersion blender, puree the soup right in the pot.
5. Spoon into bowls and enjoy warm.

Notes: I make this recipe with the skins on, but you can peel the beets if you like. You can also use a regular blender for this recipe. To do this safely, fill the blender halfway and puree the soup in batches. Leave a corner of the lid cracked or remove the top of the blender and cover it with a folded dish towel to let steam escape as you blend. Be careful not to get burned by the steam.

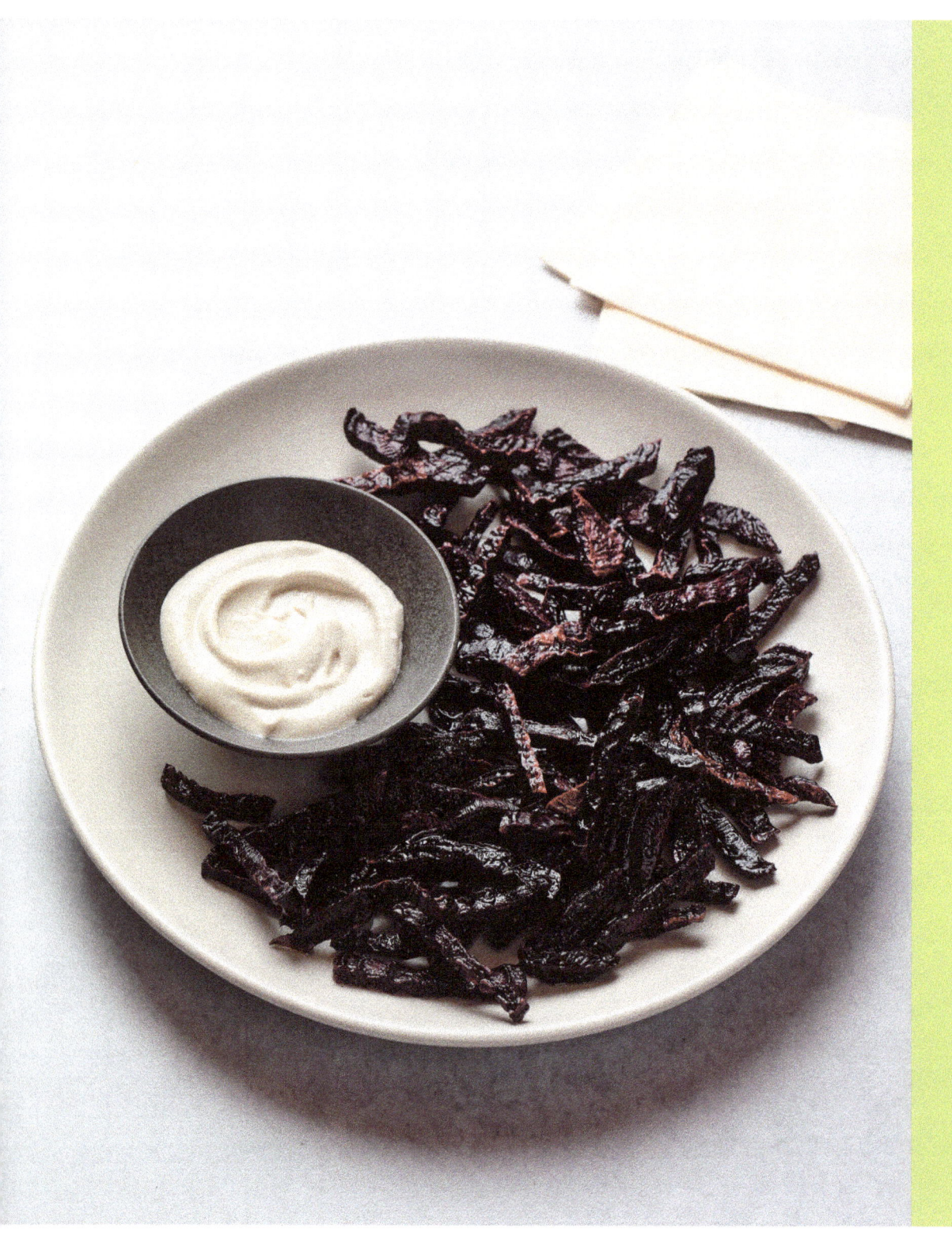

Beet Fries with Garlic Tahini

Serves 4 to 6 | Prep time: 5 minutes | Cook time: 25 minutes

These colorful fries will transform snack time at your house. Roasting beets brings out their natural sweetness, making them a delicious companion to a savory garlic tahini dip. Plus, the deep red color of beets indicates an abundance of betalains, pigments that may act as antioxidants and protect against heart disease and cell damage. These same pigments are also responsible for giving urine a harmless reddish tint after eating beets (so don't panic).

FOR THE BEET FRIES

- 3 medium beets, trimmed, peeled, and cut into ½-inch strips
- 1 tablespoon extra-virgin olive oil
- Salt

FOR THE GARLIC TAHINI

- ¼ cup tahini
- 2 garlic cloves, minced
- 1 tablespoon apple cider vinegar
- ¼ teaspoon salt

TO MAKE THE BEET FRIES

1. Preheat the oven to 400°F. Line a baking sheet with parchment paper.
2. Place the beets on the prepared baking sheet, drizzle with the olive oil, and toss until evenly coated. Sprinkle with salt.
3. Roast, flipping halfway through, for 25 to 30 minutes, or until tender.

TO MAKE THE GARLIC TAHINI

4. In a small bowl, whisk together the tahini, garlic, vinegar, and salt. Add water, 1 teaspoon at a time, whisking after each addition, until you reach your desired consistency.
5. Place the beet fries on a serving plate and serve with the dip in a small bowl on the side. Enjoy!

Notes: You can use this same method to make fries out of other root vegetables, such as carrots, parsnips, rutabaga, and sweet potatoes.

Bok Choy

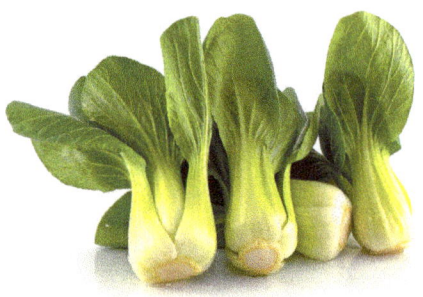

Season: Fall and Winter

Flavor profile: Also known as pak choi, this vegetable is a type of Chinese cabbage that belongs to the same family as broccoli, kale, regular cabbage, and turnips. Bok choy has tender, green leaves attached to clustered stalks and a white bulbous bottom that's crunchy and juicy. Its mild taste is more mellow than cabbage, with hints of celery.

Pairs with: Soy sauce, garlic, ginger, lemon, miso paste, hot pepper sauce, and apple cider vinegar.

Varieties: Mature (white stalks and dark green leaves) and baby (light green/white stalks and green leaves).

Preparation: Trim off the base and wash each leaf well, since dirt can hide in the stalks.

Favorite cooking methods: Halved and roasted, sautéed, and used in stir-fries.

Nutritional info: Bok choy is low in calories but very nutrient-dense. It is especially rich in the antioxidants vitamins A (carotenoids) and C and provides bone-building calcium.

Selection: Choose bok choy that has crisp leaves that are not wilted, browned, or holey. The leaves should be compact, and the stalks should be firm.

Storage: Store unwashed in a plastic bag with a few poked holes for up to 3 days in the refrigerator.

Sautéed Bok Choy

Serves 4 | Prep time: 5 minutes | Cook time: 10 minutes

Sautéed bok choy is one of the most delicious ways to prepare this green vegetable. Tender bulbs and leaves are a great match for rice or soup dishes.

1 tablespoon extra-virgin olive oil

2 garlic cloves, minced

1 teaspoon chopped fresh ginger

Pinch red pepper flakes

1 bunch bok choy, trimmed and coarsely chopped across the stems

2 tablespoons water (optional)

1. In a skillet over medium heat, warm the olive oil. Add the garlic, ginger, and red pepper flakes and cook for 1 to 2 minutes, or until fragrant.
2. Add the bok choy and cook for 3 to 5 minutes, or until the desired doneness.
3. To make the bok choy more tender, add 2 tablespoons of water, cover, and steam for another 2 to 3 minutes.

Notes: If you don't have mature bok choy, you can chop up 4 baby bok choy for this recipe.

Roasted Baby Bok Choy with Spicy Maple Miso

Serves 4 | Prep time: 5 minutes | Cook time: 10 minutes

Mellow bok choy tastes incredible with a sweet and spicy sauce. The drizzle in this recipe features sweet white miso paste made from fermented soybeans and grains. The miso contributes a creamy texture and umami flavor that elevates the entire dish. With only four main ingredients and less than 10 minutes in the oven, it doesn't get much better than this simple vegetable side.

FOR THE ROASTED BOK CHOY

- 4 heads baby bok choy, halved lengthwise, rinsed well, and dried
- 1 teaspoon extra-virgin olive oil
- Salt
- Freshly ground black pepper

FOR THE SPICY MAPLE MISO

- 1 tablespoon maple syrup
- 1 tablespoon white miso paste
- 1 teaspoon sriracha

TO MAKE THE ROASTED BOK CHOY

1. Preheat the oven to 400°F. Line a baking sheet with parchment paper. Place an oven rack in the lowest position.
2. Place the bok choy halves cut-side up on the baking sheet. Brush with half of the olive oil and season with salt and pepper. Flip over, brush with the remaining olive oil, and season with salt and pepper.
3. Roast on the lowest rack of the oven for 3 to 4 minutes. Flip the bok choy over and roast for another 3 to 4 minutes, until the leaves are wilted and slightly brown. Check frequently to ensure they don't burn.

TO MAKE THE SPICY MAPLE MISO

4. In a small bowl, mix together the maple syrup, miso, and sriracha.
5. Spoon the miso mixture over the bok choy and serve warm.

Notes: You can find miso paste at most large grocery stores in the refrigerated condiment area of the produce section or near the international aisle.

Broccoli

Season: Spring, Fall, and Winter

Flavor profile: Broccoli resembles a mini tree, with an edible stalk and a large head made up of florets. The flavor of broccoli is grassy and earthy and can be slightly bitter when raw. Roasting broccoli makes it sweeter.

Pairs with: Soy sauce, garlic, ginger, peanuts, red pepper flakes, bell peppers, and red onions.

Varieties: Belstar, Calabrese, and Destiny, as well as broccolini (see page 35).

Preparation: Rinse the head under cold running water to clean. Cut off the stalk and pull apart the florets.

Favorite cooking methods: Roasted, raw in broccoli salads, and steamed.

Nutritional info: Broccoli is a member of the cruciferous vegetable family, known for its abundance of health-promoting compounds. One of the compounds in broccoli, kaempferol, has been shown to fight inflammation and may help protect against chronic diseases. Broccoli is also rich in fiber, vitamin C, and potassium.

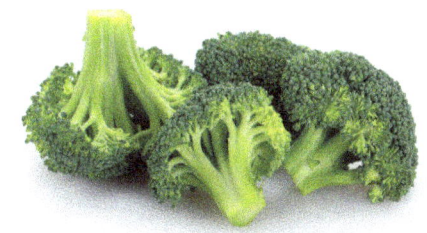

Selection: Broccoli florets should be tight and green without black or brown spots, and the stalks should appear fresh with no browning. Fresh broccoli feels heavy, even for its small size.

Storage: Keep broccoli unwashed in a loose-fitting plastic bag with some holes to allow air circulation. Store in a produce drawer in the refrigerator for up to 1 week.

Cilantro-Lime Riced Broccoli

Makes 6 cups | Prep time: 5 minutes | Cook time: 5 minutes

Move over, cauliflower rice, there's a new riced veggie in town! With the flick of a switch, you can make riced broccoli, literally, in seconds. This recipe includes a simple cilantro-lime seasoning that adds Mexican-inspired flavors. You can eat it in place of, or in addition to, regular rice for an added boost of fiber, vitamins, and minerals in bean dishes, burrito bowls, and salads.

1 head broccoli, coarsely chopped

1 tablespoon extra-virgin olive oil

2 garlic cloves, minced

2 scallions, sliced

Juice of 1 lime

2 tablespoons chopped fresh cilantro

Salt

1. In a food processor, pulse the chopped broccoli florets and stalks for 30 to 45 seconds, or until the broccoli has a rice-like texture.

2. In a large skillet over medium heat, warm the olive oil. Add the garlic, scallions, and riced broccoli and cook for 4 to 6 minutes, or until tender and warm.

3. Remove from the heat. Add the lime juice and cilantro and stir well. Season with salt.

Notes: You can also make riced broccoli by grating it, but this will take longer. Other seasoning ideas include parsley and lemon juice, or turmeric, ginger, and soy sauce.

Steamed Broccoli with Peanut Sauce

Serves 4 | Prep time: 5 minutes | Cook time: 10 minutes

Steaming vegetables is one of the simplest ways to prepare them. It helps maintain their crunch and can even preserve water-soluble nutrients. Steamed broccoli is the perfect side dish for a busy night when you need to put something on the table fast. Whip up the creamy peanut sauce while it cooks, drizzle it on top of the warm broccoli, and sit back and indulge in this unbelievably easy—and delicious—recipe.

FOR THE STEAMED BROCCOLI

2 heads broccoli, chopped into florets

FOR THE PEANUT SAUCE

¼ cup creamy peanut butter

1 tablespoon freshly squeezed lime juice

1 tablespoon rice vinegar

1 teaspoon soy sauce

½ teaspoon toasted sesame oil

1 teaspoon maple syrup

1 teaspoon chopped fresh ginger

1 garlic clove, minced

TO MAKE THE STEAMED BROCCOLI

1. Fill a large pot with 2 to 3 inches of water. Place a vegetable steamer basket inside the pot and put the broccoli florets in the basket. Bring the water to a boil over high heat. Lower the heat to medium-low, cover, and cook for 6 to 8 minutes, or until tender but still crisp.

TO MAKE THE PEANUT SAUCE

2. In a small bowl, mix together the peanut butter, lime juice, vinegar, soy sauce, sesame oil, maple syrup, ginger, and garlic. Add a few dashes of water as needed until the sauce reaches the desired consistency.

3. Add the peanut sauce to the broccoli and toss until evenly coated. Serve warm.

Notes: You can also make this recipe without a steamer basket. Just fill the pot with 1 to 2 inches of water and bring to a boil over high heat. Add the broccoli, cover, and cook for 3 to 4 minutes, or until tender. Drain before serving. You can use either fresh or frozen broccoli.

Teriyaki Tofu and Roasted Broccoli

Serves 4 | Prep time: 25 minutes | Cook time: 25 minutes

This sheet pan dinner is amazing on its own or served with rice. The tofu pairs well with the broccoli, and the zesty teriyaki sauce brings it all together. It's quick, full of flavor, and the perfect main course paired with rice.

FOR THE TOFU AND BROCCOLI

1 block extra-firm tofu

2 teaspoons low-sodium tamari or soy sauce

1½ teaspoons extra-virgin olive oil

2 teaspoons cornstarch

3 cups broccoli florets

Himalayan salt

Freshly ground black pepper

FOR THE TERIYAKI SAUCE

⅓ cup low-sodium tamari or soy sauce

3 tablespoons water

2 tablespoons maple syrup

2 tablespoons rice vinegar

1 garlic clove, grated

½ teaspoon sriracha

¼ teaspoon ground ginger

1 teaspoon cornstarch whisked together with 1 teaspoon water

1. **To make the tofu and broccoli:** Preheat the oven to 400°F. Line a baking sheet with parchment paper.
2. Drain the tofu and pat dry with paper towels. Slice the tofu into even squares. Place the tofu between two paper towels, then put something heavy on top to press out the excess water. Let sit for 15 minutes.
3. Place the pressed tofu in a mixing bowl and drizzle with the tamari and olive oil. Sprinkle on the cornstarch. Toss evenly to combine. Arrange the tofu evenly on half of the prepared baking sheet.
4. In the same mixing bowl, combine the broccoli florets, salt, and pepper. Toss together until evenly coated. Arrange the broccoli evenly on the other half of the prepared baking sheet.
5. Bake for 25 minutes, tossing the tofu and broccoli after 12 minutes.
6. **To make the teriyaki sauce:** While the broccoli and tofu bake, prepare the teriyaki sauce. In a medium saucepan over medium heat, whisk together the tamari, water, maple syrup, vinegar, garlic, sriracha, and ginger.
7. Bring the sauce to a boil, then whisk in the cornstarch mixture. Reduce the heat to low and continue to whisk until the sauce thickens.
8. Remove the tofu and broccoli from the oven and place back in the mixing bowl. Remove the teriyaki sauce from the stove and pour into the mixing bowl, coating the broccoli and tofu. Serve over brown rice.

Broccolini

Season: Spring, Fall, and Winter

Flavor profile: Broccolini is often referred to as baby broccoli, since that's exactly what it looks like, but it's actually a cross between regular broccoli and Chinese broccoli. It has longer stalks, smaller florets, and a sweeter taste compared to broccoli.

Pairs with: Soy sauce, garlic, red wine vinegar, oranges and other citrus, Italian herbs, and seasonings.

Varieties: Just one; the name broccolini is protected under a trademark.

Preparation: Rinse the head under cold running water to clean. Trim the ends with a knife.

Favorite cooking methods: Roasted, and lightly blanched.

Nutritional info: Broccolini has a nutritional profile similar to regular broccoli and other cruciferous vegetables. One cup has over 15 percent of the Daily Value (DV) for dietary fiber and provides high amounts of vitamins A and C.

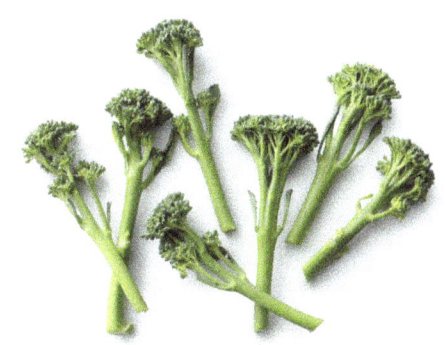

Selection: Look for broccolini with firm, moist ends that are not dried out, closed heads, and no flowers. Broccolini that has gone bad will have an unpleasant smell and yellowing around the florets.

Storage: Store broccolini in a sealed plastic bag in the refrigerator for up to 1 week. Do not wash or trim it until you plan to cook it.

Broccolini Pasta Salad

Serves 4 | Prep time: 10 minutes | Cook time: 10 minutes

Broccolini shines in this flavorful pasta salad. With every bite, you'll get hints of this sweet vegetable along with bell peppers, zesty red onion, Italian herbs, and red wine vinegar. Using broccolini instead of large broccoli florets makes the bites more manageable. This entrée or side dish is simple to prepare and makes enough for potlucks and other larger gatherings.

FOR THE PASTA SALAD

8 ounces fusilli pasta

3 cups chopped broccolini, a mix of florets and stalks

1 red bell pepper, seeded and chopped

½ cup diced red onion

FOR THE DRESSING

½ cup extra-virgin olive oil

¼ cup red wine vinegar

1 teaspoon maple syrup

1 teaspoon dried parsley

½ teaspoon dried basil

¼ teaspoon salt

TO MAKE THE PASTA SALAD

1. Bring a large pot of salted water to a boil over high heat. Add the pasta and cook for 4 to 5 minutes.

2. Add the broccolini and continue to cook the pasta and broccolini together until the broccolini is blanched and slightly tender and the pasta is al dente, 3 more minutes. Drain and rinse with cold water. Transfer to a large bowl, then add the bell pepper and onion.

TO MAKE THE DRESSING

3. In a small bowl, mix together the olive oil, vinegar, maple syrup, parsley, basil, and salt.

4. Add the dressing to the vegetables and pasta and toss until well combined.

Notes: This dish tastes even better after sitting for 30 to 60 minutes in the refrigerator. You can use Roasted Red Peppers (page 130) instead of raw and substitute penne or rotini pasta if you don't have fusilli.

Broccoli Rabe

Season: Spring, Fall, and Winter

Flavor profile: Contrary to what its name and appearance suggest, broccoli rabe (or rapini) is not a type of broccoli but is instead related to the turnip family. As a result, it has a sharp, bitter flavor. It tastes best when blanched and seasoned with garlic.

Pairs with: Olive oil, garlic, red pepper flakes, roasted red peppers, and pine nuts.

Varieties: Just one.

Preparation: Rinse under cold running water to clean. Trim the ends with a sharp knife.

Favorite cooking methods: Blanched, then sautéed; treat it similar to the way you would cook bitter greens, like turnip or mustard greens.

Nutritional info: Broccoli rabe has an impressive nutritional profile, providing high amounts of vitamins A, C, and K. It's also rich in vitamin B_5 (pantothenic acid), which aids in extracting energy

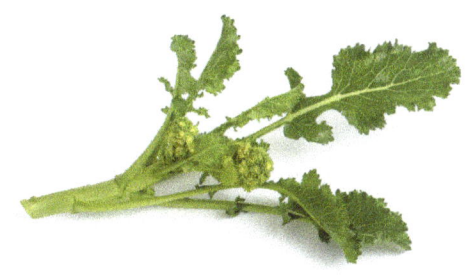

from proteins, carbohydrates, and fats in the body.

Selection: Fresh broccoli rabe has firm stalks and moist ends that are not dried out, with deep green leaves and tightly closed florets. Yellow flowers are a sign that broccoli rabe is past its prime.

Storage: Keep broccoli rabe unwashed in a sealed plastic bag in the refrigerator for up to 1 week.

Classic Sautéed Broccoli Rabe

Serves 4 | Prep time: 5 minutes | Cook time: 10 minutes

This sautéed broccoli rabe recipe is a simple, delicious, and elegant side dish to any meal. It adds the perfect variety to your traditional steamed broccoli.

1 pound broccoli rabe, trimmed and cut into 2-inch pieces

2 tablespoons extra-virgin olive oil

6 to 8 garlic cloves, minced

Pinch red pepper flakes

Salt

1. Bring a large pot of salted water to a boil over high heat. Add the broccoli rabe and cook for 2 to 3 minutes, or until blanched. Drain, rinse with cold water, and pat dry. Be careful not to overcook, or it will become mushy.

2. In a large skillet over medium-high heat, warm the olive oil. Add the garlic and red pepper flakes and sauté for 1 to 2 minutes.

3. Add the broccoli rabe and cook for 3 to 6 minutes, or until it reaches your desired doneness. Season with salt.

Notes: Store cooked broccoli rabe in more olive oil and garlic in an airtight container in the refrigerator for up to 3 days.

Brussels Sprouts

Season: Fall and Winter

Flavor profile: Raw Brussels sprouts resemble mini cabbages and have a bitter taste and tough texture. When roasted, sautéed, or steamed, Brussels sprouts are more mellow, with a slightly nutty aftertaste. Roasting Brussels sprouts brings out their natural sweetness and gives them a deliciously crispy exterior.

Pairs with: Citrus, balsamic or apple cider vinegar, mustard, sriracha or other hot pepper sauces, maple syrup, apples and apple cider, miso paste, walnuts, and pine nuts.

Varieties: Green (most common) and purple, resulting from a cross with purple cabbage.

Preparation: Remove yellow leaves and use a paring knife to cut off any small areas with holes or damage. Trim the ends and rinse the sprouts in a bowl of cold water to remove any dirt. Cut in half or use a food processor, mandoline, or knife to shred.

Favorite cooking methods: Roasted, sautéed, shaved, and shredded.

Nutritional info: Brussels sprouts are rich in fiber, vitamins C and K, and antioxidants. They also have sulfur-containing compounds known as glucosinolates that break down into isothiocyanates in the body and may exhibit anticancer effects.

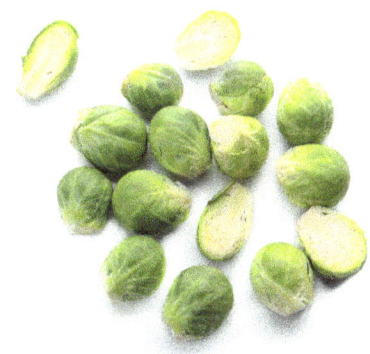

Selection: Brussels sprouts should be firm, with compact leaves that are bright green. A few yellow leaves can be normal, but avoid Brussels sprouts with withered leaves that have holes and brown spots. Some stores will sell Brussels sprouts on the stalk as well as loose.

Storage: Wait to prepare and wash Brussels sprouts until right before cooking. Store unwashed Brussels sprouts in a plastic bag or airtight container in the crisper drawer of the refrigerator for up to 1 week. Brussels sprouts on the stalk stay fresh longer, so keep them on the stalk until you are ready to prepare them.

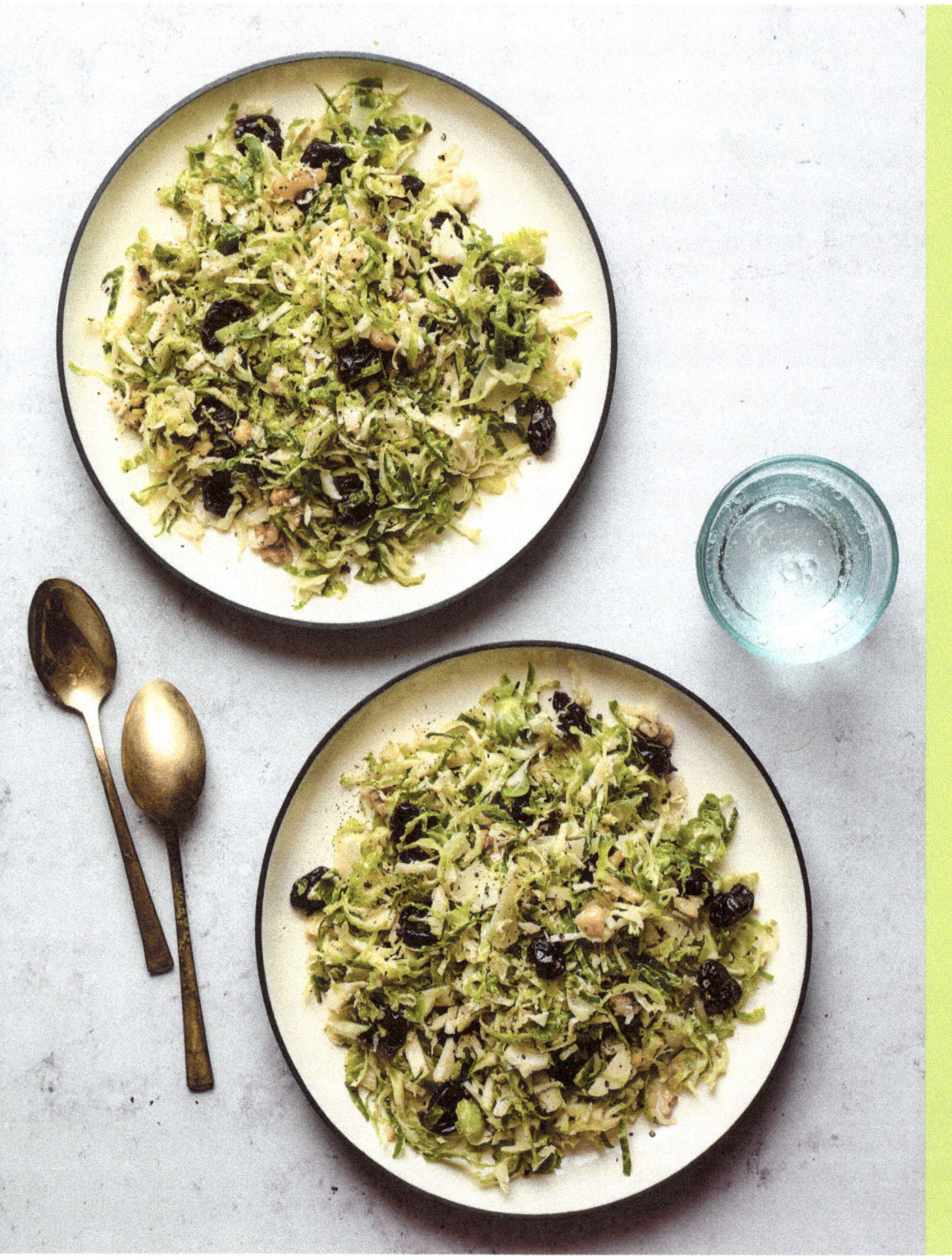

Shredded Brussels Sprouts Salad

Serves 4 | Prep time: 15 minutes

Thinly shredded Brussels sprouts are the star ingredient in this easy and delicious salad. With dried cherries, walnuts, and freshly shaved vegan Parmesan cheese, it's sweet, salty, and savory, all at the same time. Such a crowd-pleasing flavor profile makes this salad a perfect choice for holiday gatherings, meals with friends, or just a quick weeknight dinner. Add fresh seasonal fruit like apples or pears for even more fall-inspired flavor.

FOR THE SALAD

- 1 pound Brussels sprouts, trimmed
- ½ cup dried cherries
- ¼ cup chopped walnuts
- ¼ cup freshly shaved vegan Parmesan cheese

FOR THE DRESSING

- ¼ cup extra-virgin olive oil
- 3 tablespoons apple cider vinegar
- 2 teaspoons maple syrup
- 1 teaspoon Dijon mustard

TO MAKE THE SALAD

1. Shred the Brussels sprouts with a mandoline or food processor. If you don't have a mandoline, cut the Brussels sprouts in half and then into thin slices using a sharp knife.
2. Place the shredded Brussels sprouts in a large bowl and add the cherries, walnuts, and cheese.

TO MAKE THE DRESSING

3. In a small bowl, whisk together the olive oil, vinegar, maple syrup, and mustard.
4. Add the dressing to the salad and toss to combine.

Notes: You can substitute dried cranberries for the cherries, and pecans, sunflower seeds, or pine nuts for the walnuts. Several large grocery chains carry shredded Brussels sprouts in the produce section if you want to save time.

Turmeric Riced Brussels Sprouts

Makes 4 cups | Prep time: 5 minutes | Cook time: 10 minutes

Bright yellow turmeric rice is a tasty side dish that pairs well with so many main courses. This version features riced Brussels sprouts in place of traditional rice, cooked in coconut oil and anti-inflammatory ground turmeric and ginger for an extra boost of nutrition. It's delicious and colorful, and it makes a great base for salads and grain bowls.

1 pound Brussels sprouts, trimmed and halved

1 tablespoon coconut oil

½ teaspoon ground turmeric

½ teaspoon onion powder

¼ teaspoon ground ginger

Salt

Freshly ground black pepper

¼ cup raisins (optional)

1. In a food processor, pulse the Brussels sprouts for 30 to 45 seconds, or until they have a rice-like texture. You may need to do this in two batches depending on the size of your food processor.

2. In a large skillet over medium heat, warm the coconut oil. Add the Brussels sprouts, turmeric, onion powder, and ginger and cook, stirring occasionally, for 5 to 7 minutes. Season with salt and pepper.

3. Remove from the heat and stir in the raisins (if using). Serve warm.

Notes: Substitute frozen riced Brussels sprouts, available at some grocery stores, to save time. You can use 2 tablespoons of chopped fresh onion in place of the onion powder if desired.

Cabbage

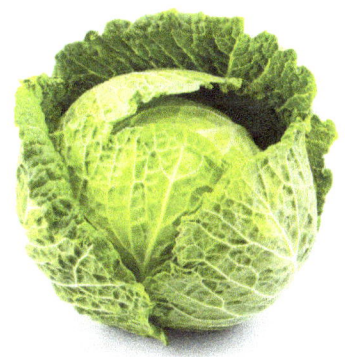

Season: Spring, Fall, and Winter

Flavor profile: While raw cabbage has a bitter taste and a tough, rubbery texture, cooked cabbage is sweeter and milder, with a buttery mouthfeel. Due to these differences, raw cabbage tastes best when it is thinly sliced and tossed with a hearty dressing. Cooked cabbage is more tender and can be enjoyed as large wedges or smaller pieces.

Pairs with: Vinegar, lime juice, peanut sauce, soy sauce, celery salt, garlic, black pepper, red pepper flakes, apples, pineapple, onions, and potatoes.

Varieties: Green, red (or purple), Napa (green, oval-shaped), and Savoy (dark green, crinkly leaves).

Preparation: Remove the outer leaves, cut in half, and wash under cold running water. Cut into quarters, then cut off the core at the bottom of each wedge before cooking or shredding into smaller pieces with a knife or mandoline.

Favorite cooking methods: Raw in salads and slaws, roasted, and braised.

Nutritional info: All cabbage varieties are low in calories, high in fiber, and rich in vitamins C and K. Red cabbage gets its color from pigments known as anthocyanins that may help decrease blood pressure and fight inflammation in the body associated with heart disease.

Selection: Choose heads of cabbage that feel heavy, with tightly packed leaves and firm stems. Wilted or discolored leaves are a sign that the cabbage is old or was mishandled.

Storage: Whole heads of cabbage can be stored in a plastic bag in the crisper drawer of the refrigerator for up to 2 weeks. Cabbage halves or quarters that have already been cut should be wrapped tightly in plastic wrap before being stored.

Braised Cabbage, Apples, and White Beans

Serves 4 | Prep time: 5 minutes | Cook time: 15 minutes

Braised cabbage shines in this hearty vegetarian main dish. Fresh apples and apple cider vinegar offer a sweet, tangy taste that beautifully complements the buttery cabbage and creamy white beans. The delicious combination of textures and flavors in this one-pan recipe, coupled with the short prep and cook time, makes it a go-to dish for weeknight meals. Plus, you can use any variety of cabbage.

2 tablespoons extra-virgin olive oil

1 small head cabbage, shredded

2 Pink Lady apples, cored and diced

¼ cup apple cider vinegar

¼ cup water

½ teaspoon salt

1 (15-ounce) can cannellini beans, drained and rinsed

1. In a large skillet over medium heat, warm the olive oil. Add the cabbage and cook for 3 to 5 minutes, or until slightly tender.
2. Add the apples and cook for another 3 to 4 minutes.
3. Add the vinegar and water and sprinkle in the salt. Reduce the heat to low, cover, and cook for 5 to 7 minutes, or until the cabbage is wilted and the apples are tender.
4. Remove the cover, stir in the white beans, and cook for 3 to 4 minutes, or until warmed through. Serve warm.

Notes: Substitute chickpeas or navy beans for the cannellini if desired. You can also use different types of apples. Store leftovers in an airtight container in the refrigerator for up to 4 days.

Quick Sesame-Soy Red Cabbage Slaw

Serves 6 | Prep time: 20 minutes

Brighten up your plate with this colorful slaw coated in a sesame-soy dressing. With fresh cilantro, ginger, and scallions, each bite packs a ton of flavor. Bring it to your next potluck, serve it alongside a stir-fry, use it as a taco topping, or bulk it up with edamame or tofu and make it a vegetarian main dish. Extra vegetables that you have on hand, like bell peppers or cucumbers, are totally fair game to add.

FOR THE SLAW

- 1 small head cabbage, shredded
- 3 scallions, thinly sliced
- 1 cup shredded carrots
- ¼ cup chopped fresh cilantro

FOR THE DRESSING

- 2 tablespoons extra-virgin olive oil
- 1 tablespoon toasted sesame oil
- 3 tablespoons rice vinegar
- 1 tablespoon soy sauce
- 2 teaspoons finely chopped fresh ginger
- 1 tablespoon maple syrup

TO MAKE THE SLAW

1. In a large bowl, mix together the cabbage, scallions, carrots, and cilantro.

TO MAKE THE DRESSING

2. In a small bowl, whisk together the olive oil, sesame oil, vinegar, soy sauce, ginger, and maple syrup.

3. Add the dressing to the slaw and toss until evenly coated. Serve right away or cover with plastic wrap and store in the refrigerator until serving.

Notes: Possible additions include 2 tablespoons of chopped fresh mint or basil, chopped peanuts, or sesame seeds. This slaw can be stored in an airtight container in the refrigerator for up to 3 days. Stir well before serving.

Carrots

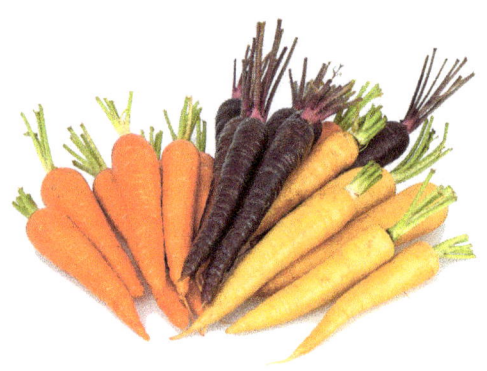

Season: Spring, Summer, Fall, and Winter

Flavor profile: One of the most universally loved vegetables, carrots have a sweet but slightly earthy flavor and a crunchy texture. Cooking carrots makes them tender and sweeter, but overdoing it can make them mushy. The pleasing taste of carrots lends itself to a wide range of dishes.

Pairs with: Savory herbs like rosemary, thyme, and dill, as well as cinnamon, nutmeg, cardamom, soy sauce, ginger, tahini, dates, maple syrup, celery, and onions.

Varieties: Orange, purple, yellow, and white.

Preparation: Remove the leaves if attached and trim the ends. Use a vegetable brush to scrub the carrots clean, or a swivel peeler to remove the outside skin. Keep them whole, cut them with a knife, or shred them with a hand grater.

Favorite cooking methods: Raw, roasted, and blended into soups and dressings.

Nutritional info: Carrots are well known for being high in beta-carotene, the pigment that gives them their orange color. In the body, beta-carotene gets converted into the antioxidant vitamin A that's vital to good eyesight, skin health, and brain function.

Selection: Fresh carrots are bright in color and have firm skin that's free of splitting or cracks. If the leaves are attached, they should be vibrant and not wilted.

Storage: Store carrots in an unsealed plastic bag in the refrigerator for at least 2 weeks or sometimes longer. Remove any greens before storing, but do not clean, trim, or cut the carrots until you are ready to cook them.

Cardamom-Maple Roasted Baby Carrots

Serves 4 | Prep time: 5 minutes | Cook time: 25 minutes

These roasted carrots have the perfect amount of flavor, and the cardamom is a great match for the natural sweetness of the carrots. The maple syrup allows them to caramelize just enough to create that perfect bite.

1 pound baby carrots, rinsed and dried

2 tablespoons extra-virgin olive oil

2 tablespoons maple syrup

¾ teaspoon ground cardamom

Salt

1. Preheat the oven to 400°F. Line a baking sheet with parchment paper.

2. Arrange the carrots in a single layer on the prepared baking sheet.

3. In a small bowl, whisk together the olive oil, maple syrup, and cardamom. Drizzle the mixture over the carrots and, using your hands or a rubber spatula, toss until they are evenly coated. Season with salt.

4. Bake for 25 to 30 minutes, or until the carrots are fork-tender. Serve hot.

Roasted Carrot and Tahini Dressing

Makes about 1 cup | Prep time: 10 minutes | Cook time: 25 minutes

Carrots are the go-to veggie to pair with dips and dressings, but they can also shine as the star ingredient of condiments. Loosely inspired by the carrot dressing sold at Trader Joe's, this tahini-based recipe is made with sweet roasted carrots and zesty ginger. It has a fibrous texture and phenomenal taste, and it makes a great addition to grain bowls and roasted vegetables like cabbage, bok choy, and broccoli.

2 cups sliced carrots

1 tablespoon extra-virgin olive oil

1 tablespoon chopped fresh ginger

1 tablespoon maple syrup

1 tablespoon soy sauce

¼ cup tahini

1. Preheat the oven to 400°F. Line a baking sheet with parchment paper.
2. Place the carrots in a single layer on the prepared baking sheet and drizzle with the olive oil. Bake for 25 to 30 minutes, or until tender.
3. Transfer the carrots to a blender. Add the ginger, maple syrup, soy sauce, and tahini and blend until smooth, using a spatula to push the mixture down the sides of the blender. Add water, 1 tablespoon at a time, to reach the desired consistency.

Notes: Store in a glass jar in the refrigerator for up to 1 week.

Salt and Vinegar Carrot Crisps

Makes about 1 cup | Prep time: 40 minutes | Cook time: 15 minutes

If you're a fan of salt and vinegar chips, you will love this vegetable-forward twist on that iconic flavor profile. After being soaked in apple cider vinegar and baked in the oven, thinly sliced carrots shrivel into small crisps that pack a ton of flavor for their size. Enjoy them on top of salads, soups, and popcorn or mixed into savory trail mixes.

Cooking spray
2 carrots
¾ cup apple cider vinegar
Salt

1. Preheat the oven to 400°F. Lightly coat two baking sheets with cooking spray.
2. Using a mandoline or a swivel peeler, thinly slice or shave the carrots. In a bowl, mix together the carrots with the vinegar and let sit for 25 to 30 minutes.
3. Using a slotted spoon or tongs, remove the carrot slices from the vinegar, place onto paper towels, and pat dry. Arrange the carrots in a single layer on the prepared baking sheet. Season liberally with salt.
4. Bake for 10 to 15 minutes, then remove any carrots that are already crispy and place them on a plate to cool. Continue to bake for another 5 to 10 minutes, or until the rest of the carrots are crispy. Watch them closely and remove pieces as they get crispy to avoid burning. Let the crisps cool at room temperature before adding more salt to taste.

Notes: These taste best when consumed within a couple of days, as they start to lose their crispiness over time. Store them in a jar at room temperature for best results.

Cauliflower and Romanesco

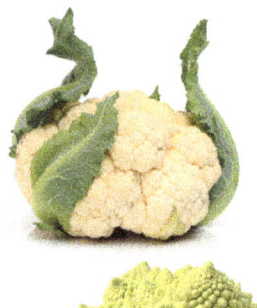

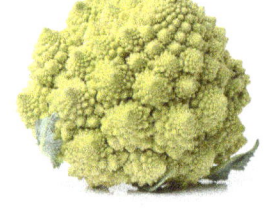

Season: Fall and Winter

Flavor profile: Cauliflower looks similar to broccoli but with white and more densely packed florets. It has a delicate flavor that's often considered nuttier and sweeter than broccoli and can easily soak up other seasonings.

Pairs with: Lemon, lime, salt, black pepper, most fresh herbs, capers, curry, red pepper flakes, hot sauces, garlic, tahini, and peanut butter.

Varieties: White, orange, and purple cauliflower. Romanesco is a type of green cauliflower (sometimes referred to as a type of broccoli) with cone-shaped florets that have a mesmerizing spiral pattern.

Preparation: Remove the leaves and cut off the bottom stem. Rinse well, upside down under cold running water, to clean. Cut into quarters, using your hands or a knife to break up the florets.

Favorite cooking methods: Processed into rice, roasted, and combined with hearty, flavorful dressings.

Nutritional info: Although it contains a variety of nutrients, cauliflower is an especially good source of vitamins C and K. It also provides choline, a mineral that's important for a healthy brain and nervous system.

Selection: Because of the white florets, it's easy to spot cauliflower that has discoloration. Look for heads that are bright white, with firm stems and no brown or black spots.

Storage: Whole heads of cauliflower can last in a perforated plastic bag in the produce drawer in the refrigerator for up to 1 week. Florets that have already been cut up should be stored in an airtight container.

Turmeric Cauliflower Steaks

Serves 4   Prep time: 5 minutes   Cook time: 25 minutes

Cauliflower steaks are juicy and mildly nutty. The turmeric adds the perfect slightly bitter flavor to this hearty vegan meal. Cut the cauliflower into thick slices to leave you feeling satiated.

1 head cauliflower

1 tablespoon extra-virgin olive oil

1 teaspoon ground turmeric

½ teaspoon garlic powder

Salt

Freshly ground black pepper

1. Preheat the oven to 400°F. Line a baking sheet with parchment paper.

2. Cut the cauliflower into 1½-inch slices lengthwise from the head through the core. Depending on the size of the cauliflower, you will get 4 to 6 flat pieces that resemble steaks. Place the slices in a single layer on the prepared baking sheet.

3. In a small bowl, mix together the olive oil, turmeric, and garlic powder. Brush the mixture onto both sides of the cauliflower steaks. Season with salt and pepper.

4. Roast, flipping halfway through the cooking time, for 25 to 30 minutes, or until tender and browned.

Spiced Cauliflower, Chickpea, and Raisin Salad

Serves 4 | Prep time: 10 minutes | Cook time: 25 minutes

This seemingly simple roasted cauliflower main dish has a complex flavor profile, thanks to cumin, cinnamon, and a lemony dressing. The chickpeas and raisins provide two additional textures that round out the whole recipe. It's a good option to prep in advance and take to work or school for lunch, especially since it can be served warm or cold.

FOR THE SALAD

- 1 head cauliflower, cut into florets
- 1 tablespoon extra-virgin olive oil
- ½ teaspoon ground cinnamon
- ½ teaspoon ground cumin
- ¼ teaspoon salt
- ¼ cup raisins
- 1 (15-ounce) can chickpeas, drained and rinsed

FOR THE DRESSING

- 3 tablespoons extra-virgin olive oil
- Juice of 1 lemon
- 2 teaspoons maple syrup
- 1 teaspoon Dijon mustard

TO MAKE THE SALAD

1. Preheat the oven to 400°F. Line a baking sheet with parchment paper.
2. Spread out the cauliflower florets in an even layer on the baking sheet. Drizzle with the olive oil.
3. In a small bowl, whisk together the cinnamon, cumin, and salt. Sprinkle the mixture over the cauliflower until evenly coated.
4. Bake for 25 to 30 minutes, or until tender.
5. Transfer the cauliflower to a large bowl, add the raisins and chickpeas, and toss.

TO MAKE THE DRESSING

6. In a small bowl, mix together the olive oil, lemon juice, maple syrup, and mustard.
7. Add the dressing to the bowl of cauliflower and toss until evenly coated.

Notes: Possible additions include chopped fresh herbs like mint or cilantro and slivered almonds.

Cauliflower Mac 'n' "Cheese"

Serves 4 | Prep time: 10 minutes | Cook time: 15 minutes

Mac and cheese is a staple in many households. This delicious vegan version is mouthwatering and full of the same creaminess you would find in the traditional recipe. The cauliflower adds just the right flavor and texture to the cream sauce. Garnish with some paprika to really bring the recipe together.

1 large head cauliflower, chopped

1 box pasta noodles

1 tablespoon extra-virgin olive oil

½ yellow onion, chopped

½ cup nutritional yeast

⅓ cup vegetable broth

1 tablespoon lemon juice

½ teaspoon garlic powder

1½ teaspoons salt

¼ teaspoon freshly ground black pepper

Smoked paprika, for garnish

1. In a large pot of boiling water, cook the cauliflower for 15 minutes, or until fork-tender. Drain.
2. While the cauliflower is cooking, cook the noodles according to the package instructions. Drain the noodles, but do not rinse.
3. While the cauliflower and pasta are cooking, warm the olive oil in a medium saucepan over medium-low heat. Add the onions and cook for 10 minutes.
4. In a high-speed blender, blend the cauliflower, onions, nutritional yeast, broth, lemon juice, garlic powder, salt, and pepper until smooth.
5. In a large bowl, combine the noodles with the sauce. Stir to coat evenly. Garnish with the paprika.

Celery

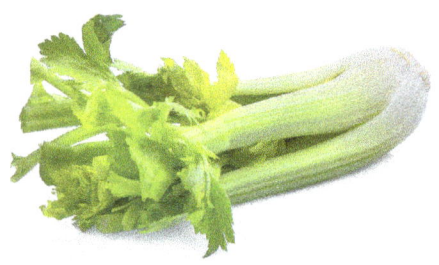

Season: Spring, Summer, and Fall

Flavor profile: Known for its distinct stringy texture, celery has an earthy, mineral-like taste. To some, celery has a salty aftertaste, as a result of its relatively higher natural sodium content compared to other vegetables.

Pairs with: Citrus, nut butters, dried fruit, buffalo and hot sauce, carrots, and onions.

Varieties: Celery (thicker stalks) and leaf celery (thinner stalks, with aromatic leaves).

Preparation: Separate each stalk from the bunch and trim off the bottoms and tops. Wash the stalks under cold running water, using your hands to rub off any dirt. Use a sharp knife to cut the stalks into the desired size pieces. Remove and discard any leaves, or keep them to add to dishes as garnish.

Favorite cooking methods: Raw and stuffed, and cooked into sauces and soups.

Nutritional info: Celery is well known for being low in calories and mostly made of water. However, it also provides fiber, antioxidants, and a compound called apiuman that may help strengthen the stomach lining and prevent stomach ulcers.

Selection: Look for firm stalks and light green leaves, and avoid celery that appears wilted, soggy, or dried out. It should feel crisp and not rubbery to the touch.

Storage: Wrapping celery in aluminum foil helps prevent moisture from leaking out and will keep it from getting mushy and limp. Store it in the produce drawer in the refrigerator for up to 1 week. Celery that has already been cut should be submerged in water in an airtight container and kept in the refrigerator.

Celery with Almond Butter and Pomegranate Arils

Serves 4 | Prep time: 5 minutes

You can't go wrong with this healthy snack, a simple classic. The almond butter adds a delicious flavor and is a change from peanut butter, which is commonly used. Additionally, the pomegranate arils, which are the juice-packed seeds of the fruit, add a layer of tangy sweetness to cut through the creamy nut butter.

8 celery stalks, cut into 3-inch pieces

4 tablespoons almond butter

2 tablespoons pomegranate arils

Cinnamon, for serving

Using a butter knife or spoon, stuff each celery piece with almond butter. Press the pomegranate arils into the almond butter, sprinkle with cinnamon to taste, and serve.

Celery Root

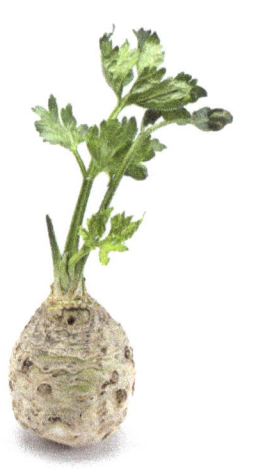

Season: Fall and Winter

Flavor profile: Celery root, also known as celeriac, is a knobby root vegetable with potato-like white flesh and brown skin that's studded with bumps and ridges. As a relative of classic celery, it has a similar taste that's milder, with nutty undertones.

Pairs with: Apples, lemon, garlic, onions, potatoes, and mustard.

Varieties: Just one.

Preparation: Trim the ends and use a swivel peeler to remove the skin. For skin stuck in the ridges, use a paring knife to make small cuts to remove the skin. Dice before roasting, boiling, or sautéing.

Favorite cooking methods: Roasted, mashed, and blended into soups.

Nutritional info: Celery root is loaded with vitamins and minerals but is low in carbohydrates, making it a good alternative to potatoes for those watching their carb intake. It's particularly rich in fat-soluble vitamin K and, thus, may support healthy blood clotting.

Selection: To choose fresh celery root, make sure it is firm to the touch, with brown skin. It's normal to see a few hints of green around the top of the vegetable where the stalks were removed, but this should not be widespread. If the stalks are still attached, make sure they are firm and have fresh leaves.

Storage: Keep in a perforated plastic bag in the produce drawer in the refrigerator for up to 2 weeks.

Garlicky Celery Root and Potato Soup

Serves 4 | Prep time: 10 minutes | Cook time: 30 minutes

Made with two hearty root vegetables and a roasted garlic bulb, this simple but flavorful soup is a great way to warm up in the winter. Plus, it's a no-waste recipe, because not only will you use celery root for the mellow, earthy flavor that makes up the base of the soup, but you can also save the stalks and leaves to use as garnish.

1 tablespoon extra-virgin olive oil

1 yellow onion, diced

1 large celery root, peeled and diced

1 russet potato, peeled and diced

4 cups vegetable broth

Salt

Freshly ground black pepper

1 Roasted Garlic Bulb (page 82)

Celery root stalks and leaves, chopped, for garnish

1. In a large stockpot or Dutch oven over high heat, warm the olive oil. Add the onion and sauté for 3 to 4 minutes.

2. Add the celery root, potato, and broth and bring the mixture to a boil. Lower the heat to medium-low, cover, and cook for 20 to 25 minutes, or until the vegetables are tender.

3. Remove the pot from the heat, season with salt and pepper, and squeeze the roasted garlic cloves out of the bulb and into the soup. Stir well. Using an immersion blender, puree the soup. Taste and season with salt and pepper as desired.

4. Ladle into bowls and garnish with chopped celery root stalks and/or leaves. Serve hot.

Notes: If you have celery root that does not have its stalks, serve the soup with another fresh herb (like chopped fresh chives or parsley) instead. To blend the soup safely in a regular blender, fill it halfway and puree the soup in batches. Leave a corner of the lid cracked, or remove the top of the blender and cover it with a folded dish towel to let steam escape as you blend. Be careful not to get burned by the steam.

Chard

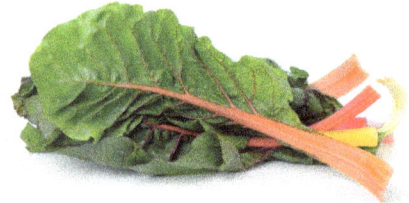

Season: Spring, Fall, and Winter

Flavor profile: Chard leaves are earthy and slightly bittersweet, with a taste similar to spinach and beets. They are firm and tough, but less so than kale and collards. All parts of chard are edible, and some consider the stems to be sweeter than the leaves.

Pairs with: Onions, garlic, red wine and balsamic vinegars, lemon, red pepper flakes, maple syrup, and mint.

Varieties: Swiss chard (all green) and rainbow chard (yellow, red, white, and orange stalks and stems).

Preparation: Rinse the leaves under cold running water and pat dry with clean towels. Use a sharp knife to remove the leaves from the center stem, then cut the leaves into strips and chop the stems.

Favorite cooking methods: Raw, sautéed, and mixed into eggs, salads, and grain dishes for color and flavor.

Nutritional info: Chard is rich in potassium, magnesium, and calcium, three nutrients that play a pivotal role in maintaining healthy blood pressure. It also provides fiber and high amounts of vitamins A and K.

Selection: Chard leaves should be vibrant and dark green with bright stems. They should not be wilted, and the stems should not look dried out. To test whether chard is fresh, rub your fingers on a leaf to determine whether it is still firm and smooth.

Storage: The best way to store chard is in a plastic bag in the refrigerator for up to 1 week. Be sure to squeeze out as much air as possible before sealing the bag for best results.

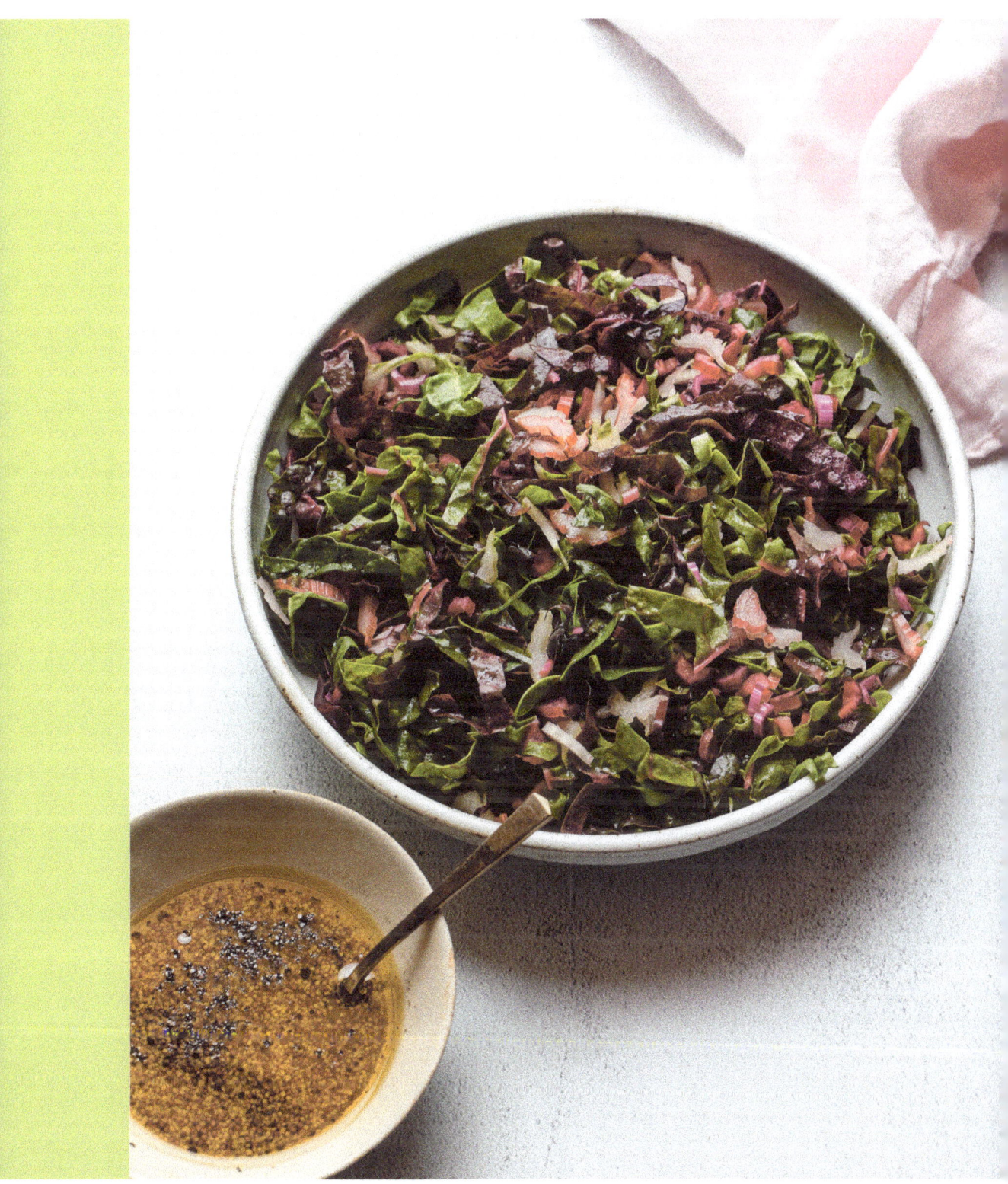

Maple Chard Salad, p. 60

Maple Chard Salad

Serves 4 | Prep time: 5 minutes

This chard salad is full of natural sweetness from the maple syrup. The perfect go-to salad.

- 3 tablespoons extra-virgin olive oil
- 2 tablespoons apple cider vinegar
- 2 tablespoons maple syrup
- 2 teaspoons whole-grain mustard
- 1 bunch chard, cut into strips and stems chopped

1. In a small bowl, whisk together the olive oil, vinegar, maple syrup, and mustard.
2. In a large bowl, combine the dressing with the chard and toss until evenly coated.

Chicories

Season: Fall and Winter

Flavor profile: The chicory family includes a variety of colorful, leafy vegetables that look similar to lettuce. They generally have a bittersweet taste, with escarole and frisée being less bitter than radicchio and Belgian endive. Unless you are particularly fond of this taste, it's best to pair chicories with ingredients that subdue their bitterness and bring out a softer flavor.

Pairs with: Citrus, balsamic vinegar, red or white wine vinegars, dried fruit, garlic, onions, and sweeteners.

Varieties: Radicchio (dark purple/red leaves with white veins), escarole (green, looks similar to romaine lettuce), frisée (thin, "frizzy" leaves that are green and yellow), and Belgian endive (see page 73).

Preparation: Best techniques depend on the specific chicory, but you can wash all varieties under cold running water to clean. Use a sharp knife to trim off the ends and chop as desired.

Favorite cooking methods: Raw, sautéed, and roasted.

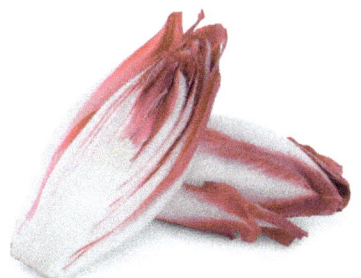

Nutritional info: Chicories are generally low in calories and provide an abundance of vitamins and minerals. Most varieties are high in vitamin K, and some are also rich in folate and vitamins A and C.

Selection: As when selecting any leafy vegetable, look for heads with fresh leaves that are not wilted or discolored.

Storage: Loosely wrap escarole, radicchio, or frisée in a damp paper towel and keep in a plastic bag in the refrigerator to use within a few days.

Escarole and White Bean Soup

Serves 4 | Prep time: 5 minutes | Cook time: 20 minutes

Escarole and white beans are a common culinary pair, but I wasn't aware of how delicious they could be together until I tasted them in soup form. The bittersweet flavor of escarole is perfectly complemented by creamy white beans, garlic, and red pepper flakes in this healthy recipe. With such a short cook time and ingredients list, this soup will become a new favorite in no time.

- 1 tablespoon extra-virgin olive oil
- 1 yellow onion, diced
- 4 garlic cloves, minced
- 1 tablespoon fresh thyme
- ¼ teaspoon red pepper flakes
- Salt
- Freshly ground black pepper
- 1 head escarole, coarsely chopped
- 4 cups vegetable broth
- 1 (15-ounce) can cannellini beans, drained and rinsed
- Freshly grated vegan Parmesan cheese, for serving (optional)

1. In a large pot or Dutch oven over medium heat, warm the olive oil. Add the onion, garlic, thyme, and red pepper flakes and season with salt and pepper. Cook for about 5 minutes.
2. Add the escarole, broth, and beans and stir to combine. Bring the soup to a gentle boil, stirring occasionally, and cook for 15 minutes. Using the back of a wooden spoon, mash about half of the beans in the pot. This makes the soup creamier and helps it thicken up.
3. Serve with freshly grated cheese if desired.

Notes: If you have one on hand, add a small Parmesan rind to the soup while it cooks for even more flavor. Remove before eating. Other possible additions include fresh lemon juice and crusty bread for serving.

Corn

Season: Summer

Flavor profile: Corn has a sweet taste and a soft, buttery texture, although the flavor profile can be more or less sweet depending on the variety. Raw corn tends to be starchier and less sweet than cooked.

Pairs with: Salt, fresh herbs, peppers, chili powder, potatoes, stone fruit, tomatoes, farro, and rice.

Varieties: Sweet corn, dent or field corn (used for animal feed and industrial corn products), and flint corn (hard kernels in a variety of colors, mostly ornamental).

Preparation: Remove the husks and underlying strings that may get stuck on the cob. Trim off the ends with a sharp knife if cooking whole, or use a serrated knife to easily cut off the kernels.

Favorite cooking methods: Boiled, grilled, and raw.

Nutritional info: In addition to being high in fiber and B vitamins, corn provides a variety of beneficial plant compounds. Two of these compounds, lutein and zeaxanthin, make up a large part of the eye and promote proper eye health.

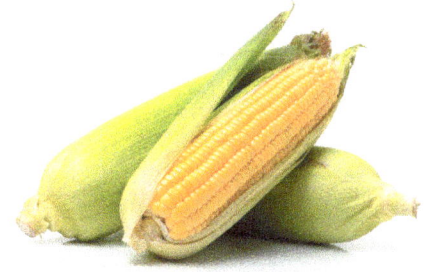

Selection: The husks of fresh corn are tightly wrapped around the cob and should feel slightly moist. While you may think that brown or sticky strings at the top of the husks (the tassel) is a bad sign, this is normal. But if the tassel is black, dry, or mushy, the corn is likely old.

Storage: Store corn in the husks in a sealed plastic bag in the produce drawer in the refrigerator. Use within a few days.

Corn Chowder

Serves 4 | Prep time: 15 minutes | Cook time: 50 minutes

Corn chowder is highly underrated. With potatoes, vegan butter, and coconut milk, this version is sure to please anyone. The sweetness of the corn and the creaminess of the coconut milk create a delicious soup base, and you can eat this as a main course or as a side.

5 corn cobs

3 tablespoons vegan butter

1 yellow onion, chopped

1 teaspoon crushed garlic

1 teaspoon dried thyme

½ cup gluten-free flour

2 cups vegetable broth

2 (13.5-ounce) cans coconut milk

2 large potatoes, peeled and cubed

1 bay leaf

¾ cup chopped spring onions, plus more for serving

1 teaspoon Himalayan salt

Freshly ground black pepper

1. Slice all the corn off the cobs. Break or cut the cobs in half and set aside.
2. In a large pot, melt the butter. Add the yellow onion and sauté for 7 minutes, or until soft.
3. Add the garlic and thyme and cook for 5 minutes.
4. Stir in the flour, broth, and coconut milk and cook for 5 minutes.
5. Add the corn cobs, potatoes, and bay leaf. Bring to a simmer, cover, and cook for 20 minutes, or until the potatoes are soft.
6. Remove and discard the corn cobs and the bay leaf. Add the fresh corn and cook for 10 minutes.
7. Stir in the spring onions. Add the salt and sprinkle on some pepper to taste.
8. Serve with some more spring onions on top and a sprinkle of pepper.

Fresh Corn and Cherry Dip

Makes about 4 cups | Prep time: 15 minutes

The fresh flavors in this corn and cherry dip are a perfect match for tortilla chips, but you can also serve it on top of grilled summer squash for a light side dish. It's colorful, nutritious, and fun, and it makes a great addition to a warm-weather cookout or Fourth of July spread. Depending on where you live, cherry and corn seasons may overlap for a short (and magical) period of time. But if you can't find one of the main ingredients fresh, frozen or canned varieties work just as well.

2 cups fresh sweet corn kernels

2 cups cherries, pitted and thinly sliced

½ cup diced red onion

2 tablespoons chiffonaded fresh basil

2 tablespoons chopped fresh mint

Juice of 1 lemon

Salt

Combine the corn, cherries, onion, basil, mint, and lemon juice in a medium bowl and stir well. Taste, and add salt as desired. Serve with tortilla or pita chips.

Notes: To remove the pits of fresh cherries, insert a reusable stainless steel straw into the center of each cherry to gently pop out the pit.

Cucumbers

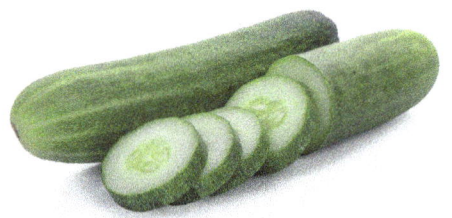

Season: Summer

Flavor profile: Cucumbers have a distinct crispness with a light, slightly sweet flavor that can sometimes be bitter. Their taste may also be described as hydrating, since they have a high water content and fairly juicy flesh.

Pairs with: Onions, tomatoes, fresh fruit, vinegar, citrus, dill, and black pepper.

Varieties: Garden cucumbers (large seeds), English cucumbers (seedless), pickling (Kirby) cucumbers, and gherkins (very small).

Preparation: Wash cucumbers under cold running water, using your hands or a vegetable brush to rub the skin clean. Use a swivel peeler to remove the skin if desired. To remove the seeds, cut into quarters lengthwise and then make a thin slice down the center of each quarter to slice off the seeds.

Favorite cooking methods: Raw, and pickled.

Nutritional info: Cucumbers are over 96 percent water and can help contribute to daily water intake. They provide vitamins C and K, potassium, manganese, and several compounds that may act as antioxidants and prevent damage to cells in the body.

Selection: Choose cucumbers that are firm, with bright green skin free of blemishes or indications of rotting.

Storage: Wrap cucumbers tightly with plastic wrap, or place them in paper towels in a sealed plastic bag. Store in the produce drawer in the refrigerator for up to 1 week.

Spicy Cucumber, Cashew, and Edamame Salad

Serves 4 | Prep time: 15 minutes

The refreshing, cool taste of cucumbers, coupled with their crunchy texture, makes them an ideal counterpart to a spicy dressing. Chopped cashews add a nutty undertone and a source of healthy fats, and edamame contributes plant-based protein. This balanced dish can be served as a main or side and is a good option to prep in advance for lunch.

FOR THE SALAD

1 large cucumber, peeled, seeded, and diced

¾ cup cooked edamame

½ cup chopped dry-roasted cashews

2 tablespoons chopped fresh cilantro

FOR THE DRESSING

2 tablespoons sriracha

1 tablespoon extra-virgin olive oil

1 tablespoon rice vinegar

1 teaspoon maple syrup

2 garlic cloves, minced

TO MAKE THE SALAD

1. In a medium bowl, mix together the cucumber, edamame, cashews, and cilantro.

TO MAKE THE DRESSING

2. In a small bowl, whisk together the sriracha, olive oil, vinegar, maple syrup, and garlic.

3. Add the dressing to the salad and toss until evenly coated. Taste and adjust the seasonings as desired.

Notes: Store in the refrigerator in an airtight container for up to 5 days. Possible additions include sesame seeds, chopped fresh mint, or a squeeze of lime juice.

Cucumber-Melon Salsa

Makes about 4 cups | Prep time: 15 minutes

Cucumbers are a headliner vegetable (well, technically a fruit) of summer. Many home gardeners find themselves swimming in cukes by the middle of the season. If you find yourself in that pickle (pun intended), this sweet yet spicy salsa is for you. Made with cucumber and cantaloupe in place of tomatoes, it's a wonderfully fresh and colorful snack. Pair it with tortilla chips for an afternoon treat, or serve it over grilled vegetables and tofu.

1 garden cucumber, peeled and diced

½ cantaloupe, seeded and diced

½ cup chopped red onion

1 jalapeño pepper, seeded and finely chopped

Juice of 1 lemon

2 tablespoons chopped fresh cilantro, plus more as needed

1 tablespoon extra-virgin olive oil

Salt

Freshly ground black pepper

In a medium bowl, mix together the cucumber, cantaloupe, red onion, and jalapeño. Add the lemon juice, cilantro, and olive oil and stir well. Season with salt and pepper, and add more cilantro to taste.

Notes: You can serve this immediately with tortilla or pita chips, but it tastes especially delicious after sitting in the refrigerator for about 1 hour to let the flavors meld.

Eggplant

Season: Summer

Flavor profile: Eggplants, also known as aubergines, have deep purple skin with tan flesh that has brown spots surrounding the seeds. Known for its spongy texture, eggplant can soak up flavors very well. However, its taste alone is bland and slightly bitter.

Pairs with: Onions, tomatoes, zucchini, bell peppers, basil, oregano, parsley, garlic, and soy sauce.

Varieties: Globe (big and plump), Japanese (thin and long), Rosa Bianca (purple-and-white-streaked skin), and white.

Preparation: To reduce the bitterness of its flesh, eggplant slices are often sprinkled with salt and left to sit until they begin to "sweat." This practice helps draw out moisture and any unpleasant tastes along with it.

Favorite cooking methods: Grilled, sautéed or braised, roasted, and breaded.

Nutritional info: Eggplants offer vitamins, minerals, and fiber, but they also contain anthocyanin pigments that are responsible for their colorful skin. Consumption of anthocyanins has been associated with possible anti-cancer effects.

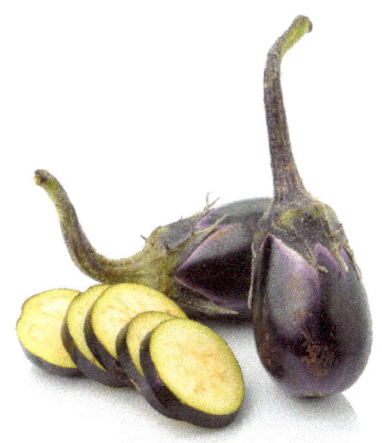

Selection: To test the freshness of an eggplant, press your thumb into the skin to ensure that it is firm and not squishy. Inspect the skin and choose shiny eggplants that do not have bruises.

Storage: Fresh eggplant is best stored at room temperature in a cool, dry area that does not get direct sunlight. Keep it away from bananas and melons, or transfer it to a plastic bag and keep in the refrigerator.

Eggplant Bacon

Serves 6 | Prep time: 10 minutes | Cook time: 20 minutes

This plant-based twist on bacon offers a similar smoky and salty flavor profile and makes a great addition to vegetarian BLTs and breakfast sandwiches. If you want to take it a step further and mimic the crispiness of true bacon, cut the eggplant as thin as possible. I even went so far as to pull out a ruler to help me make perfect 1/16-inch slices, and it made all the difference. A mandoline can come in handy for this recipe but is not required.

- 4 tablespoons extra-virgin olive oil, divided
- 2 tablespoons soy sauce
- 1 tablespoon maple syrup
- 1 teaspoon vegan smoked paprika
- 1 teaspoon vegan Worcestershire sauce
- 1 medium eggplant, cut into 1/16-inch slices

1. In a small bowl, whisk together 2 tablespoons of olive oil and the soy sauce, maple syrup, smoked paprika, and Worcestershire sauce. Brush each slice of eggplant on both sides with the mixture and transfer to a plate.

2. In a large skillet over medium heat, warm the remaining 2 tablespoons of olive oil until fragrant. Place the eggplant slices in a single layer in the skillet and cook, gently flipping with tongs, for 4 to 5 minutes on each side, or until slightly charred and crispy. (You will likely have to cook them in batches.) Keep a close eye on the eggplant to make sure the slices don't burn. The next batches will take less time as the skillet heats up.

3. Transfer the eggplant to a plate lined with paper towels. The eggplant will continue to crisp up as it cools. Enjoy immediately.

Notes: This recipe is definitely crispiest when eaten right away, but it can be stored in an airtight container in the refrigerator for up to 3 days. Use tamari in place of soy sauce to make this gluten-free, and be sure to use a vegan Worcestershire sauce if you want or need it to be vegan.

Eggplant Parmesan

Serves 2 | Prep time: 15 minutes | Cook time: 40 minutes

Delicious roasted eggplant replaces the lasagna noodles in this classic recipe, giving it an extra nutritional boost. The vegan mozzarella can be found in the plant-based section at your local grocery store and makes this dish taste very authentic.

2 medium eggplants, trimmed and cut into ½-inch slices

Pinch kosher salt

Pinch freshly ground black pepper

½ cup panko bread crumbs

½ cup grated vegan Parmesan cheese

½ cup fresh basil, chopped, plus more for serving

1 tablespoon Italian seasoning

3½ cups marinara sauce

16 ounces vegan mozzarella

1. Preheat the oven to 400°F. Line a large baking sheet with parchment paper.
2. Place the eggplant slices on the baking sheet and sprinkle with the salt and pepper. Roast for 15 minutes, flip the eggplant slices, and continue to bake for another 15 minutes.
3. In a small bowl, combine the bread crumbs, Parmesan, basil, and Italian seasoning, tossing evenly to coat.
4. Once the eggplant is done baking, remove it from the oven and reduce the heat to 375°F.
5. Ladle ½ cup of the marinara sauce into a 9-by-9-inch baking dish. Arrange a third of the eggplant on top of the sauce in the baking dish. Cover the eggplant with a third of the mozzarella. Add half the remaining sauce, then add another third of the eggplant, and cover the eggplant with another third of the mozzarella. Add one more layer of eggplant, top it with the rest of the sauce, and finish with the last third of the mozzarella.
6. Sprinkle the bread crumb topping evenly over the top of the dish.
7. Cover with foil and bake for 10 minutes. Garnish with chopped fresh basil, if desired, and serve.

Japanese Eggplant with Thai Basil

Serves 2 | Prep time: 10 minutes | Cook time: 20 minutes

This eggplant dish is savory, zesty, and spicy. The Thai basil, which is very different from traditional basil, brings a fresh taste. Japanese eggplant is much smaller than regular eggplant, and it works like a charm for soaking up the delicious sauce.

FOR THE SAUCE

2½ tablespoons maple syrup

3 tablespoons tamari

2 tablespoons rice vinegar

2 teaspoons sriracha

1 teaspoon toasted sesame oil

Pinch ground coriander

Pinch ground cinnamon

⅓ cup water

FOR THE EGGPLANT

4 tablespoons avocado oil

½ large red bell pepper, sliced

½ large green bell pepper, sliced

½ medium yellow onion, sliced

2 medium Japanese eggplants, cut into even slices

5 garlic cloves, minced

1 (1½-inch) piece fresh ginger, chopped

1 Thai green chile, sliced

2 teaspoons cornstarch mixed with 2 tablespoons water

Himalayan salt

½ cup Thai basil, chopped, plus more for garnish

TO MAKE THE SAUCE

1. In a blender or food processor, blend the maple syrup, tamari, vinegar, sriracha, sesame oil, coriander, cinnamon, and water until smooth.

TO MAKE THE EGGPLANT

2. In a medium pan over medium heat, warm the avocado oil. Add the red and green bell peppers, onion, eggplants, garlic, and ginger and cook for 10 minutes, stirring frequently.

3. Add the chile and continue to cook for another 3 minutes.

4. Slowly pour in the sauce and the cornstarch mixture, then stir until it thickens.

5. Mix together evenly, cover, and let simmer for 7 minutes. Season with salt.

6. Garnish with the basil and serve.

Notes: Pair this dish with jasmine rice for a wonderful combination.

Endive

Season: Fall and Winter

Flavor profile: Belgian endive has a cylindrical shape, with narrow, tightly packed leaves, a white base, and either yellow or purple-red tips. A type of chicory, it has a crunchy texture and subtle bitterness that can be mellowed by cooking methods and flavor pairings.

Pairs with: Citrus, dried fruit, apples, garlic, sunflower seeds, and pistachios.

Varieties: Just one, but they can have yellow or red leaves.

Preparation: Trim off the end and cut in half or into thin slices. If you intend to keep the leaves whole, separate them with your hands.

Favorite cooking methods: Braised, and raw.

Nutritional info: Belgian endive is rich in fiber that can promote optimal digestion. It's also a good source of bone-strengthening vitamin K.

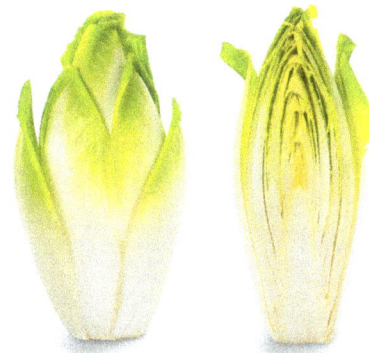

Selection: Endive leaves should cling together and appear firm. Discolored or wilted leaf tips are an indication that the vegetable is old and has almost gone bad.

Storage: Since endive likes the dark, wrap it in paper towels before placing it in a plastic bag to store in the refrigerator. It can last in the produce drawer for up to 1 week and sometimes a bit longer.

Braised Endive

Serves 4 | Prep time: 5 minutes | Cook time: 30 minutes

This slow-cooked recipe turns the endives into tender, luscious, and mildly sweet bundles. Each endive is juicy and dripping with flavor, making it the perfect side to any rice or potato dish.

2 tablespoons extra-virgin olive oil

4 to 6 heads Belgian endive, trimmed

Juice of 1 lemon

½ cup vegetable broth

5 or 6 thyme sprigs

In a pot or Dutch oven over medium heat, warm the olive oil. Place the whole endives into the pot, nestling them together in a single layer. Squeeze the lemon juice over the top, pour in the broth, and add the thyme sprigs. Reduce the heat to low, cover, and simmer for about 30 minutes, or until tender.

Fava Beans

Season: Spring

Flavor profile: Fava beans, also known as broad beans, come in large green pods. The beans are removed from their pods before cooking and eating. When properly prepared, they have a buttery and slightly nutty taste that's often described as spring-like.

Pairs with: Peas, artichokes, mint, tomatoes, onions, garlic, olive oil, salt, and most nuts.

Varieties: Can vary in shape, size, and color.

Preparation: Break open the bean pods to remove the beans. To get rid of the waxy coating, blanch the beans in boiling water for 30 to 60 seconds and transfer them to an ice bath. The coating will be easy to peel off after this process. One pound of bean pods yields about 1 cup of peeled beans.

Favorite cooking methods: Steamed, mashed, and added to salads or pasta.

Nutritional info: Fava beans are packed with plant-based protein and contain a high amount of folate, a water-soluble vitamin that's especially important for pregnant women to consume to prevent birth defects.

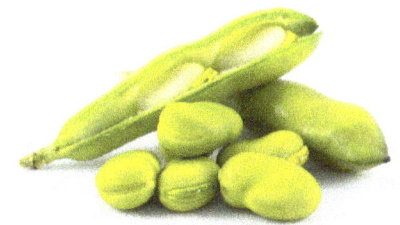

Selection: Choose broad beans that have smooth, bright green pods. You should be able to see bumps from the beans inside, but they should not be bulging, as this may be an indicator that they are old.

Storage: Store fava beans still in their pods in a paper or plastic bag in the refrigerator for up to 10 days. Shelled fava beans can be stored in the freezer for up to 3 months.

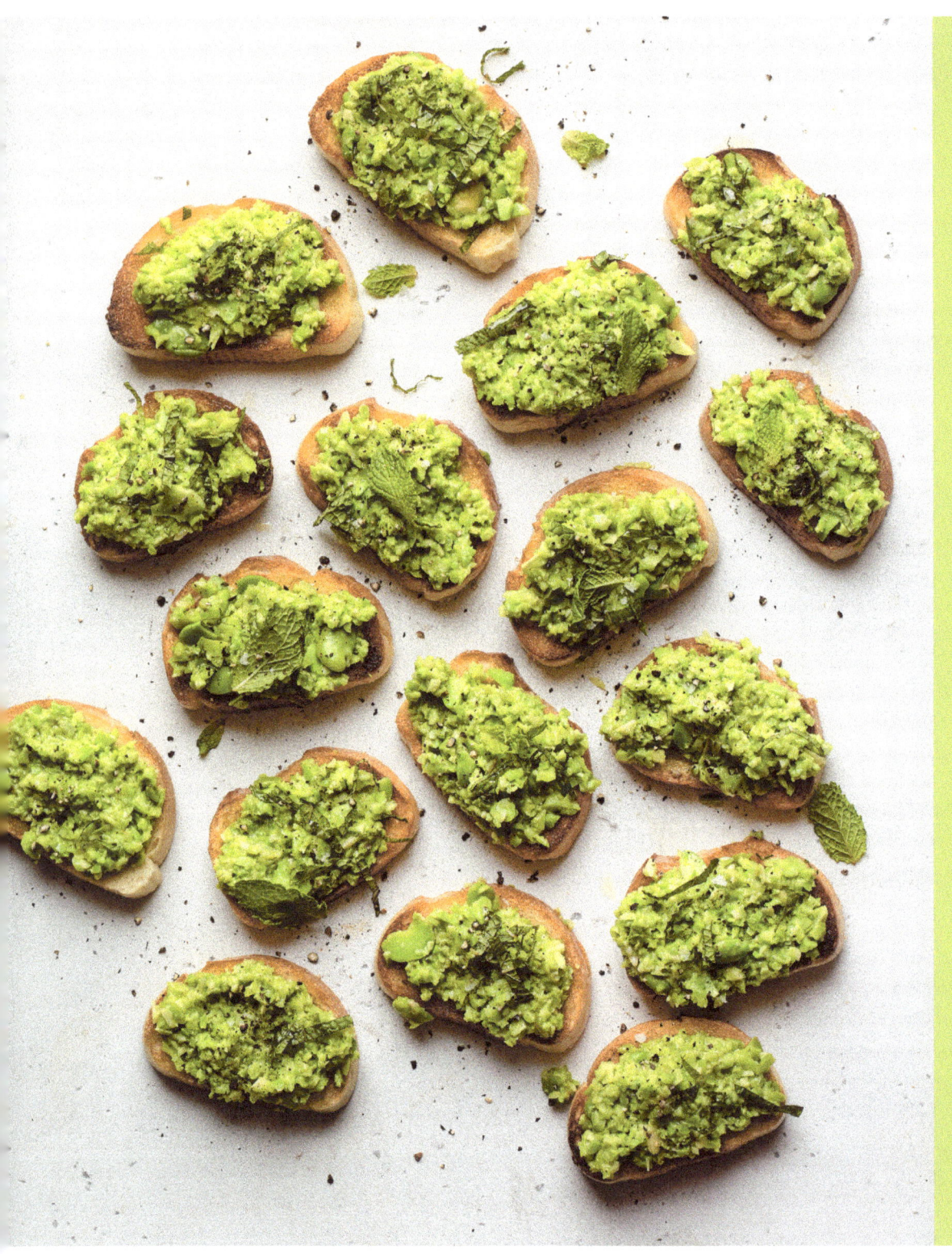

Mashed Fava Bean Bruschetta

Serves 6 | Prep time: 15 minutes | Cook time: 5 minutes

Vegetal fava beans shine in this spring-inspired bruschetta, complemented by garlic, fresh mint, and lemon. Although the preparation of these beans can be tedious, the mashed fava beans are lusciously creamy and delicious. Make a batch of marinated fava beans a few days in advance so that they have time to soak up the flavors before you prepare this recipe.

12 (½-inch) slices Italian bread or baguette

1 tablespoon extra-virgin olive oil

2 garlic cloves, minced

Marinated Fava Beans (page 78)

Juice of 1 lemon

¼ cup chopped fresh mint

Salt

Freshly ground black pepper

1. Turn the broiler on high.
2. Place the bread slices on a baking sheet. In a small bowl, mix together the olive oil and garlic. Brush the mixture onto the bread. Broil for 2 to 3 minutes, or until lightly toasted.
3. Transfer the fava beans to a bowl using a slotted spoon. Squeeze in the lemon juice and mash the beans with a fork. Depending on how tender the beans are, they will be more or less difficult to mash. For a creamier mash, pulse the beans in a food processor with the lemon juice instead.
4. Spread a spoonful of the fava mash on the toasted bread. Top with the mint and season with salt and pepper.

Notes: Possible additions include red pepper flakes and fresh basil.

Marinated Fava Beans

Makes about 1 cup | Prep time: 15 minutes, plus 24 hours to marinate | Cook time: 1 minute

Fava beans are sweet, tender, and pleasantly starchy. This recipe is vegan, versatile, and delicious! Use these on toast, bruschetta, or salads.

1 pound fava bean pods
¼ cup red wine vinegar
¼ cup extra-virgin olive oil
2 tablespoons chopped fresh parsley
2 garlic cloves, minced
½ teaspoon salt
¼ teaspoon red pepper flakes

1. Bring a pot of salted water to a boil over high heat. Break open each bean pod to remove the beans. Drop the beans into the boiling water and blanch for 30 to 60 seconds. Immediately drain the beans and submerge them in a bowl with ice water. The process of blanching ensures that the beans stay green and fresh. Drain the beans again and use your fingers to squeeze each bean and remove the skin.

2. In a 1-pint glass jar, combine the vinegar, olive oil, parsley, garlic, salt, and red pepper flakes and shake well. Place the fava beans in the jar, seal tightly, and shake to combine. Refrigerate for at least 24 hours before serving.

Fennel

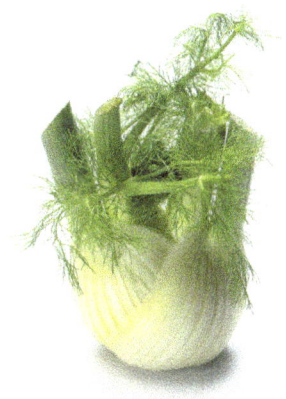

Season: Fall and Winter

Flavor profile: Fennel is a bulbous vegetable with a white base, bright green stalks, and wispy fronds. While all parts of fennel are edible, typically only the base is used in recipes. It has an anise-like taste that contributes a sweet and subtle licorice flavor to dishes.

Pairs with: Tomatoes, garlic, onions, carrots, beets, oranges, lemons, Granny Smith apples, red wine vinegar, red pepper flakes, and hazelnuts.

Varieties: Herb fennel (cultivated for its stems, leaves, and seeds) and Florence fennel (grown for its bulb to be eaten as a vegetable).

Preparation: Cut off the stalks, fronds, and ends. Cut the bulb into quarters and remove the core at the bottom of each quarter with a paring or chef's knife.

Favorite cooking methods: Raw, roasted, braised, and seared.

Nutritional info: In addition to being a good source of fiber and vitamin C, fennel provides manganese. This trace mineral is important for metabolism and blood sugar regulation.

Selection: The freshest fennel bulbs are white without any brown spots or bruises. If the stalks and fronds are attached, make sure they look vibrant and do not have any flowers.

Storage: Before storing, trim fennel stalks about 2 inches above the bulb. Keep the bulbs in a sealed plastic bag in the refrigerator for about 1 week.

Roasted Fennel and Tomatoes over Pasta

Serves 6 | Prep time: 10 minutes | Cook time: 30 minutes

With their tender texture, flavorful juices, and mouthwatering caramelization, roasted tomatoes are one of my favorite foods. Pairing them with fennel, which gets just as caramelized through roasting, brings this recipe to a whole new level. Be sure to line your baking sheet with foil so that you can easily funnel the tomato and fennel juices onto your plate for maximum flavor. If you find yourself eating the whole tray, don't say I didn't warn you of its deliciousness.

2 pounds cherry tomatoes, halved

1 fennel bulb, thinly sliced

½ sweet onion, thinly sliced

3 tablespoons extra-virgin olive oil

½ teaspoon dried basil

¼ teaspoon dried oregano

Salt

Freshly ground black pepper

6 cups cooked pasta, for serving

1. Preheat the oven to 450°F. Line a baking sheet with aluminum foil.

2. Place the tomatoes, fennel, and onion on the prepared baking sheet. Drizzle with the olive oil, and sprinkle with the basil and oregano. Season with salt and pepper. Using your hands or a rubber spatula, toss the mixture until evenly coated. The baking sheet will be a little crowded, but that's okay.

3. Roast for 30 to 40 minutes, or until the fennel is tender and the tomatoes are caramelized. Serve warm over the pasta.

Notes: You can use 1 teaspoon each of chopped fresh basil and oregano instead of dried if available. Add the basil after roasting. For more protein, mix in white beans or chickpeas.

Garlic

Season: Summer and Fall

Flavor profile: Although it is typically considered a seasoning by chefs and home cooks alike, garlic is a vegetable by botanical definition. Garlic bulbs pack several cloves that provide a spicy, strong, sinus-clearing taste that's reminiscent of garlic's relatives: onions, shallots, leeks, and chives.

Pairs with: Olive oil, most vinegars, citrus, soy sauce, ginger, red pepper flakes, rosemary, thyme, oregano, and most fresh herbs.

Varieties: Softnecks (no scape, smaller in size, white skin) and Hardnecks (scape, can have purple stripes on skin). Garlic scapes are also harvested during the summer and can be used in cooking.

Preparation: Break off the number of cloves you need from the bulb with your hands or with the help of a paring knife. Smash each clove with the side of the blade of a chef's knife or use a silicone garlic roller to help remove the skin. You can then use a garlic press or knife to mince the cloves.

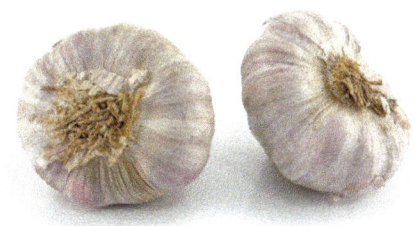

Favorite cooking methods: Minced and added as a seasoning, and roasted whole.

Nutritional info: Garlic contains a variety of compounds that have been linked to immune-boosting health benefits, lower blood pressure, and a decreased risk of heart disease.

Selection: Choose bulbs that are firm, without any green shoots sprouting out of the center. There should be no areas that are dark or dried out.

Storage: Store whole garlic bulbs at room temperature in a cool, dry area or in a garlic keeper.

Roasted Garlic Bulbs

Makes 2 bulbs | Prep time: 5 minutes | Cook time: 30 minutes

Roasting whole garlic bulbs is an easy and delicious method. The sweet, soft cloves can be used in countless ways. The classic way to enjoy these caramelized cloves is to simply spread them on crusty bread with a little sprinkle of salt and eat as is.

2 garlic bulbs

2 tablespoons extra-virgin olive oil

1. Preheat the oven to 400°F.
2. Remove most of the papery skin surrounding the garlic bulbs, but leave the skin on individual cloves so that the bulb remains intact. Using a sharp knife, cut ½ inch off the top of the cloves. Place each bulb on a square of aluminum foil. Drizzle 1 tablespoon of olive oil onto the cloves of each bulb, using your fingers to rub it over the cut surfaces. Wrap the bulbs in the aluminum foil.
3. Roast for 30 to 40 minutes, or until the bulbs feel soft. Let cool. Using a spoon, remove the roasted cloves or squeeze them out with your fingers.

Notes: Spread the roasted garlic on bread or add to dressings and marinades.

All-Purpose Garlic Marinade

Makes about ½ cup | Prep time: 5 minutes

Garlic on its own is an incredibly versatile seasoning that can be used in countless ways. But it's nice to have a go-to garlic marinade that's tried and true. This basic recipe features fresh lime juice and mustard that provides just enough zest and tang to complement the garlic. You can also modify it with ingredients you have on hand, such as lemon juice or apple cider vinegar instead of lime juice.

¼ cup extra-virgin olive oil

Juice of 2 limes

4 garlic cloves, minced

2 tablespoons whole-grain mustard

½ teaspoon salt

½ teaspoon freshly ground black pepper

In a glass jar with a lid, combine the olive oil, lime juice, garlic, mustard, salt, and pepper. Seal the lid and shake well. Use as a salad dressing or to marinate vegetables before grilling.

Notes: Store in a jar in the refrigerator for up to 2 weeks. Shake well before using.

Ginger

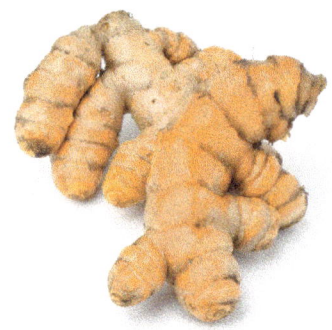

Season: Fall

Flavor profile: Ginger, as most home chefs know it, is the bumpy root of a flowering plant that's commonly used as a spice in cooking. Although it's not technically a vegetable, it's vital to preparing flavorful vegetarian meals. It has a strong, spicy taste.

Pairs with: Sesame, soy sauce, garlic, peanut butter and peanuts, lime juice, rice vinegar, apple cider vinegar, sugar, molasses, and autumnal spices.

Varieties: Several, but the most commonly consumed have brown skin and yellow flesh.

Preparation: Fresh ginger root should be peeled before using. You can use a spoon, a swivel peeler, or a knife to remove the skin.

Favorite cooking methods: Minced or grated and added to marinades and dressings, candied, and used in baked goods.

Nutritional info: Ginger is widely used as a home remedy for nausea. It has also been shown to fight inflammation and, therefore, is added to many dishes and products for an anti-inflammatory boost.

Storage: Unpeeled ginger root can be stored in a sealed plastic bag in the refrigerator for 2 to 3 weeks. Wrap any cut surfaces with plastic wrap before storing.

Homemade Candied Ginger

Makes about 4 cups | Prep time: 10 minutes, plus 3 hours to dry | Cook time: 50 minutes

As someone who suffers from motion sickness, I use ginger as a natural antiemetic anytime I fly or get on a boat, typically in the form of candied ginger. My frequent consumption of this treat helped me realize its variety of culinary uses in baked goods, salads, and roasted vegetables. Instead of purchasing expensive candied ginger at the store, you can actually make it right in your own kitchen.

- 1 pound ginger, peeled and thinly sliced with a mandoline
- 2 cups granulated sugar, plus more for dusting

1. Place a wire rack over a baking sheet.
2. Place the ginger in a saucepan and add just enough water to cover. Bring the mixture to a boil over high heat. Lower the heat to medium, cover, and cook for about 20 minutes. Drain the ginger, reserving ¼ cup of liquid.
3. Add the ginger and the reserved ginger water back to the saucepan and add the sugar. Bring to a boil over high heat, stirring well. Lower the heat to medium and cook, stirring occasionally, until the ginger appears almost dry and the sugar is about to recrystallize, 30 to 40 minutes. Immediately remove from the heat. Using a slotted spoon, transfer the ginger to the wire rack.
4. Let the ginger dry out for at least 3 hours before tossing it in more granulated sugar to taste.

Note: If you have a candy thermometer, it should read 225°F when the ginger is ready to be removed from the heat. Candied ginger can be stored in a tightly sealed jar or a zip-top plastic bag at room temperature for up to 4 weeks.

Green Beans

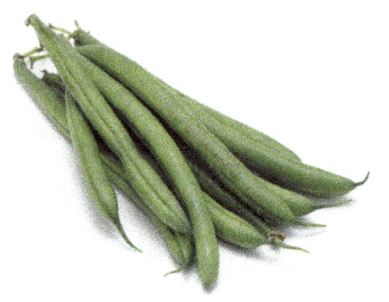

Season: Summer and Fall

Flavor profile: The bright green color of fresh green beans is a good indicator of their slightly sweet, grassy flavor. Their subtle taste makes them a versatile option for side dishes and salads. Plus, they add a delicious crunch to any recipe.

Pairs with: Red onions, garlic, basil, parsley, thyme, cayenne pepper, paprika, soy sauce, ginger, white beans, and almonds.

Varieties: Green beans (also known as string beans), haricot verts (French green beans, thinner), purple string beans, and yellow wax beans.

Preparation: Trim green beans by snapping off the ends with your fingers or using a knife.

Favorite cooking methods: Blanched, sautéed, and roasted.

Nutritional info: Green beans are low in calories but rich in fiber and micronutrients. They are a good source of immune-boosting vitamin C, providing over 25 percent of the Daily Value (DV) per cup.

Selection: Look for green beans that are bright and crisp and snap easily. They should not have any dark spots or rotting.

Storage: Place green beans in a sealed plastic bag or an airtight container in the refrigerator for up to 1 week.

Blackened Green Beans

Serves 4 | Prep time: 5 minutes | Cook time: 10 minutes

These easy and super flavorful green beans are smothered in blackening seasoning made from a base of paprika, garlic powder, oregano, basil, and cayenne pepper. They're inspired by the delicious blackened green beans on the menu at Grace Tavern in the Fitler Square neighborhood of Philadelphia, where I first tried this style of green beans several years ago. Serve this easy side dish with almost any entrée for the ultimate flavor boost (and sinus clearing!).

4 tablespoons extra-virgin olive oil, divided

1 teaspoon smoked paprika

½ teaspoon dried oregano

½ teaspoon garlic powder

½ teaspoon freshly ground black pepper

¼ teaspoon salt

¼ teaspoon dried basil

⅛ teaspoon cayenne pepper

1 pound green beans, trimmed

1. In a large bowl, whisk 2 tablespoons of olive oil and the paprika, oregano, garlic powder, black pepper, salt, basil, and cayenne pepper. Add the green beans and toss until evenly coated.

2. In a large skillet over medium heat, warm the remaining 2 tablespoons of olive oil. Add the green beans and cook, stirring occasionally, for 5 to 8 minutes, or until tender.

Notes: You can also roast the green beans. Line a baking sheet with parchment paper. Spread the beans out in a single layer on the baking sheet and roast at 400°F for 15 to 20 minutes, or until tender.

Green Beans and Potatoes

Serves 2 | Prep time: 10 minutes | Cook time: 25 minutes

In this one-pan dinner that's big on flavor, the soft potatoes mixed with the green beans and vegetable broth will have you feeling full and satisfied. It's an ultra-comforting recipe that can be served as a main dish or a side.

3 cups potatoes, peeled and sliced

4 cups fresh or frozen green beans

½ teaspoon dried thyme

¼ teaspoon freshly ground black pepper

1 teaspoon vegan Worcestershire sauce

1 cup vegetable broth, divided

1 teaspoon cornstarch

¼ cup chopped parsley, plus more for garnish

1. In a large skillet over medium-high heat, combine the potatoes, green beans, thyme, pepper, Worcestershire sauce, and ¾ cup of broth. Bring to a boil. Reduce the heat to low, cover, and simmer for 20 minutes, or until the vegetables are tender.

2. In a small bowl, combine the remaining ¼ cup of broth and the cornstarch. Stir in the parsley and add to the potato mixture.

3. Cook, stirring, until bubbly and thickened. Serve garnished with fresh parsley.

Herbs

Season: Spring, Summer, and Fall

Flavor profile: Herbs are truly one of the most important groups of seasonings for flavorful, plant-forward cooking. Each herb offers a unique flavor profile, ranging from the cool, sweet taste of fresh mint to the woody, piney notes found in rosemary.

Pairs with: Dressings, marinades, and all vegetables.

Varieties: Rosemary, basil, thyme, oregano, mint, parsley, cilantro, dill, tarragon, sage, and chives.

Preparation: Wash most herbs under cold running water to clean. Some recipes call for whole leaves, while others require chopped herbs.

Favorite cooking methods: Used as seasonings, mixed into dressings and condiments, and dried.

Nutritional info: While the exact nutritional benefits of every herb are unclear, it's thought that adding herbs to foods generally has a positive effect on health.

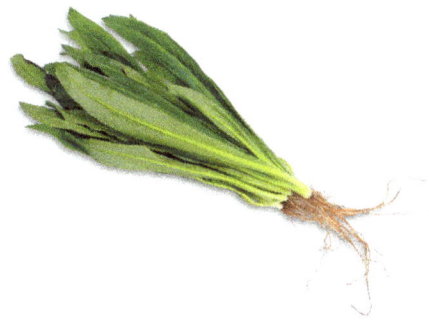

Selection: Herbs should have bright-colored leaves that are not wilted or mushy.

Storage: Most herbs can be kept for up to 1 week. Store fresh basil upright in a glass jar with water, covered loosely with a plastic bag, at room temperature away from direct sunlight. Rosemary, thyme, and oregano should be wrapped in a paper towel inside a plastic bag in the refrigerator. Parsley, cilantro, and mint can be stored upright in glass jars filled with water in the refrigerator. For the best storage results, change the water your herbs are in every 2 to 3 days.

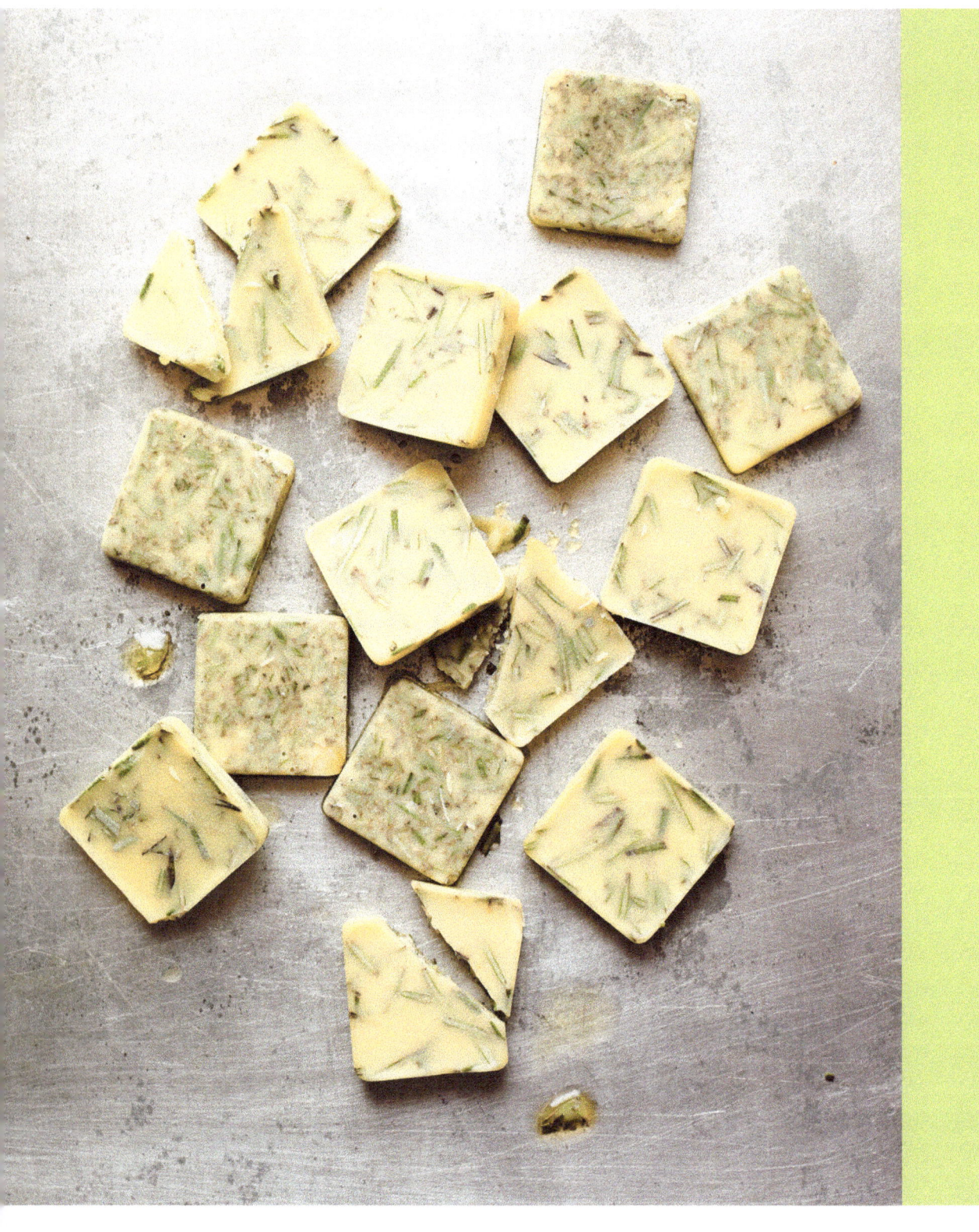

Frozen Olive Oil and Rosemary Cubes

Makes 12 cubes | Prep time: 5 minutes, plus 4 hours to freeze

Fresh rosemary is known for its piney flavor and strong fragrance. It pairs wonderfully with fall and winter vegetables, including beets, parsnips, carrots, winter squash, and other root vegetables. If you grow rosemary in your summer garden and want to preserve it for colder months, making frozen olive oil and rosemary cubes is the way to go. You can enjoy the delicious flavors of fresh rosemary all year long with the help of this freezer recipe.

1 cup chopped fresh rosemary

¾ cup extra-virgin olive oil, plus more as needed

1. Divide the chopped rosemary equally between the cubes in a 12-cube ice cube tray. Add enough olive oil to just barely cover the herbs. Each cube typically contains about 1 tablespoon of olive oil and a little more than 1 tablespoon of rosemary.

2. Freeze for at least 4 hours. Gently pop the cubes out of the tray and store them in a sealed and labeled zip-top plastic bag in the freezer for use later. When you want to use one, simply add to it to the skillet or pot you are using.

Notes: You can use this same method for all different kinds of herbs.

DIY Dried Herbs

A fun and easy DIY project at home. Transform herbs into a culinary staple by simply drying them at home. Store in glass jars on your spice rack.

Herbs of choice, such as thyme, rosemary, oregano, or sage

If you are harvesting your own herbs, cut them from your garden just before drying. Rinse the herbs under cold running water to clean. Pat dry with paper towels. Combine 5 to 10 branches together for each herb. Tie them together with twine or string, and hang them upside down by the string from a hook, a curtain rod, or another platform in a warm room in your home. Some herbs take 1 to 2 weeks to dry, while others may take longer. The herbs are properly dried when they look shriveled and brown and feel crunchy when rubbed with your fingers. Store dried herbs in small airtight containers for use later.

Homemade Chimichurri

Makes about 1 cup | Prep time: 10 minutes

Chimichurri is a vibrant green sauce made from fresh parsley and cilantro that's popular in South American and Mexican cooking. While it's typically served with meat and fish, it's also a delicious addition to plant-based recipes. You can serve it on top of cauliflower or kohlrabi steaks or use it as a dipping sauce for veggie chips and fries.

- 1 cup loosely packed fresh parsley leaves (about 1 bunch)
- 1 cup loosely packed fresh cilantro leaves (about 1 bunch)
- 4 garlic cloves, minced
- ½ cup extra-virgin olive oil
- ¼ cup red wine vinegar
- ½ teaspoon salt
- ¼ teaspoon freshly ground black pepper
- ¼ teaspoon red pepper flakes

In a food processor, combine the parsley, cilantro, and garlic, and pulse once or twice. Add the olive oil, vinegar, salt, black pepper, and red pepper flakes, and pulse until smooth, using a rubber spatula to scrape down the sides as needed.

Notes: Store in an airtight container in the refrigerator for up to 7 days.

Jicama

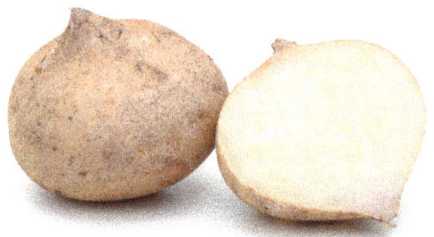

Season: Fall and Winter

Flavor profile: Native to Mexico, jicama is a type of tuber with brown skin and white flesh that resembles a potato. It has a crunchy texture, similar to an apple, and a sweet, nutty taste.

Pairs with: Lime juice, chili powder, cilantro, dill, parsley, red wine vinegar, fresh fruit, and soy sauce.

Varieties: Several, but they look similar.

Preparation: Peel jicama with a swivel peeler, then use a knife to cut it into desired shapes.

Favorite cooking methods: Raw, spiralized, riced, and roasted.

Nutritional info: Jicama packs over 6 grams of fiber in just one cup. It is particularly rich in prebiotic fiber that feeds gut bacteria, contributing to a healthy microbiome.

Selection: Fresh jicama is firm to the touch and has smooth skin that should not appear dry. Smaller jicama are thought to have a sweeter taste.

Storage: Whole jicama can be stored at room temperature in a cool, dry place for up to 2 weeks or sometimes a little longer. Once it has been peeled and cut, keep it in a sealed plastic bag or airtight container in the refrigerator for up to 1 week.

Baked Jicama Fries with Homemade Chimichurri

Serves about 4 | Prep time: 5 minutes | Cook time: 30 minutes

These jicama fries have the perfect crispy fry texture. Enjoy this healthier take on fries that are higher in fiber, lower in carbs, and a perfect match for your favorite dipping sauce.

1 large jicama, peeled and cut into ½-inch strips

1 tablespoon extra-virgin olive oil

½ teaspoon garlic powder

Homemade Chimichurri (page 93), for dipping

1. Preheat the oven to 400°F. Line a baking sheet with parchment paper.
2. Arrange the jicama fries in a single layer on the baking sheet. Drizzle with the olive oil and sprinkle with the garlic powder. Using your hands or a rubber spatula, toss until evenly coated.
3. Bake, flipping halfway through, for 30 to 35 minutes, or until tender and slightly browned. Enjoy warm with chimichurri or another dipping sauce of your choice.

Jicama-Mango Salsa

Makes about 6 cups | Prep time: 15 minutes, plus 1 hour to chill

Or should I say Jica-mango Salsa? This hydrating, juicy snack is the perfect way to cool off on a hot summer's day. It's crunchy, fruity, spicy, and refreshing all at the same time, with simple ingredients to boot. I like eating it with tortilla chips, but I've also found myself enjoying it straight out of the jar with a spoon. You can serve this salsa on grilled vegetable steaks or spooned over roasted zucchini in the summer.

1 medium jicama, peeled and cubed

1 mango, peeled and cubed

½ cup chopped red onion

1 jalapeño, seeded and finely chopped

2 tablespoons chopped fresh cilantro

2 tablespoons chopped fresh dill

Juice of 1 lime

Salt

In a medium bowl, mix together the jicama, mango, onion, jalapeño, cilantro, and dill. Squeeze the lime juice over the top and season with salt. Chill for at least 1 hour to allow the flavors to meld together before serving, or enjoy immediately if you just can't wait.

Kale, Collards, and Other Greens

Season: Spring, Fall, and Winter

Flavor profile: Kale is a hearty leafy green vegetable with a tough texture and an earthy taste. Its flavor is stronger than that of spinach and more similar to other greens with robust tastes like collards, chard, and beet greens.

Pairs with: Vinegars, citrus, garlic, olive oil, raisins, dried cranberries, coconut, apples, pecans, and walnuts.

Varieties: Kale can be green or purple in color. The most common varieties are curly kale and lacinato (dinosaur) kale. Other leafy greens include turnip, beet, mustard, collard, arugula (see page 14), bok choy (see page 28), chard (see page 58), spinach (see page 145), and watercress.

Preparation: Use your hands or a knife to remove leaves from the stems. Rinse thoroughly under cold running water to clean. Pat dry. To soften, massage it in your hands with a drizzle of olive oil.

Favorite cooking methods: Raw in salads, braised, and blended into smoothies.

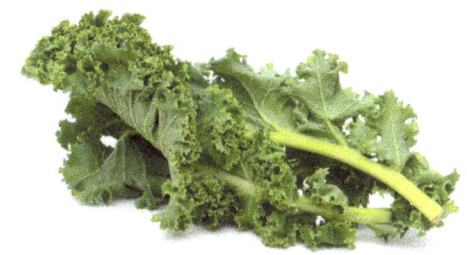

Nutritional info: Kale and most other hearty greens are incredibly rich in the antioxidant vitamins A and C. One cup of kale also provides close to 700 percent of the Daily Value (DV) of vitamin K, a fat-soluble vitamin that's necessary for proper blood clotting.

Selection: Kale and similar leafy green vegetables should have a bright color, without dark spots or holes. The leaves should not be wilted or yellow, and the stems should not be dried out.

Storage: Store leafy greens unwashed between paper towels in a sealed plastic bag in the produce drawer of the refrigerator. They typically last for 1 week.

Coconut Braised Kale

Serves 4 | Prep time: 5 minutes | Cook time: 10 minutes

This kale recipe is rich, juicy, savory, and sweet all at once. The kale is cooked down so it's as soft as butter and can be enjoyed simply with a side of rice.

1 (13.5-ounce) can full-fat coconut milk

1 tablespoon soy sauce

Juice of 1 lime

1 bay leaf

Pinch red pepper flakes

1 bunch kale, stemmed and coarsely chopped

Salt

In a large skillet over medium heat, combine the coconut milk, soy sauce, lime juice, bay leaf, and red pepper flakes. Add the kale and cook, stirring occasionally, until tender, 10 to 12 minutes. Remove and discard the bay leaf. Season with salt.

Crispy Kale Chips

Serves 4 | Prep time: 10 minutes | Cook time: 25 minutes

Satisfy your afternoon cravings with these salty, crispy, and savory kale chips—the perfect snack food. It's easy to "eat your greens" with this recipe, especially when you're not in the mood for a salad. Just remember to follow the directions closely and avoid overcrowding your baking sheets to ensure that the chips get as crispy as possible.

1 bunch curly kale, stemmed and roughly torn

1 or 2 tablespoons extra-virgin olive oil

1 teaspoon garlic powder

Salt

Freshly ground black pepper

1. Preheat the oven to 300°F. Line two baking sheets with parchment paper.
2. Wash the kale under cold running water and pat dry with paper towels. Make sure that the kale is completely dry, since any leftover moisture on the leaves will steam them while cooking and make the chips soggy.
3. Divide the kale equally between the two baking sheets. Drizzle with enough olive oil to lightly coat the leaves and use your hands to toss them. Spread the leaves out in a single layer without any overlapping. Sprinkle with the garlic powder, and season with salt and pepper.
4. Bake for 10 minutes, rotate the baking sheets, and bake for another 15 minutes, or until the chips are slightly browned and crispy.

Notes: Other possible seasoning combinations include 1 teaspoon chili powder with ½ teaspoon paprika and ½ teaspoon garlic powder. For "cheesy" chips, mix 2 tablespoons nutritional yeast with 1 teaspoon garlic powder and salt to taste.

Sautéed Mustard Greens

Serves 4 | Prep time: 5 minutes | Cook time: 15 minutes

When cooked down in a skillet with a few simple ingredients, the peppery taste of mustard greens shines. They make a delicious, simple, and interesting side dish next to any entrée, and they deliver a ton of vitamin K and other nutrients at the same time. Substitute any hearty leafy green, including turnip, beet, and radish greens that would otherwise go to waste.

1 tablespoon extra-virgin olive oil

3 garlic cloves, minced

1 bunch mustard greens, chopped

Salt

Freshly ground black pepper

¼ cup vegetable broth

1. In a large skillet over medium heat, warm the olive oil. Add the garlic and cook, stirring frequently, for about 1 minute, or until fragrant.
2. Stir in the greens and cook until just wilted. Season with salt and pepper.
3. Add the broth, bring to a simmer, and cook for another 3 to 4 minutes. Serve warm.

Notes: For a different flavor profile, add 1 teaspoon of toasted sesame oil and a pinch of red pepper flakes to the pan with the olive oil and garlic.

Gumbo Z'Herbes

Serves 4 | Prep time: 20 minutes | Cook time: 50 minutes

The traditional version of this vegan gumbo is usually eaten on Good Friday, but this take on it is so packed with healthy leafy greens and loaded with flavorful veggies that you won't miss the meat. The legend behind this dish is that the more greens you add, the more luck you'll have.

⅓ cup vegan butter

⅔ cup all-purpose flour

2 green bell peppers, diced

2 celery stalks, finely chopped

1 yellow onion, diced

2 cups vegetable broth

1 head cauliflower, cut into florets

1 cup cremini mushrooms, sliced

3 garlic cloves, minced

1 tablespoon Cajun seasoning

½ teaspoon liquid smoke

1 bay leaf

1 (15-ounce) can fire-roasted peppers

1 (15-ounce) can kidney beans, drained and rinsed

½ cup kale, chopped

1 cup mustard greens, chopped

1 cup collard greens, chopped

½ teaspoon Himalayan salt

½ teaspoon freshly ground black pepper

Chopped spring onions, for garnish

1. In a large pan, melt the butter over medium heat. Slowly mix in the flour and stir to create a paste. Keep stirring for about 20 minutes, or until it changes to a thin sauce. Be careful not to burn the flour.

2. When the flour mixture turns into a thin sauce, add the bell peppers, celery, and onion. Continue to cook until the vegetables are soft.

3. Slowly pour in the broth and stir to combine. Add the cauliflower florets, mushrooms, garlic, Cajun seasoning, liquid smoke, bay leaf, fire-roasted peppers, and kidney beans and stir to combine. Bring to a simmer, cover, and simmer for 30 minutes, or until everything is cooked and fragrant.

4. Add the kale, mustard greens, collard greens, salt, and pepper. Stir to combine.

5. Remove and discard the bay leaf. Garnish with chopped spring onions and serve.

Notes: This recipe goes well with basmati rice.

Kohlrabi

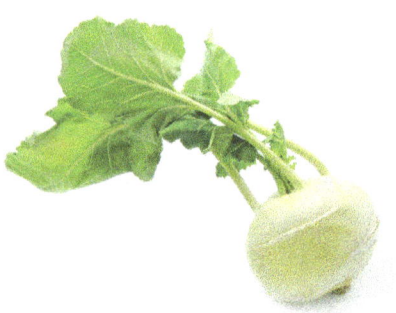

Season: Spring, Fall, and Winter

Flavor profile: Kohlrabi is a bulbous vegetable related to cabbage and turnips. It has stalks with leaves that shoot out of its skin in different areas, but typically only the bulb is eaten. The taste of kohlrabi is very similar to broccoli stems, but older kohlrabi can taste closer to turnips.

Pairs with: Thyme, rosemary, oregano, chives, dill, basil, tomatoes, lemon, carrots, potatoes, sesame, ginger, and mustard.

Varieties: Green or purple.

Preparation: Remove the stalks and peel with a swivel peeler or a knife. Use a sharp knife to dice or cut into steaks. Kohlrabi also lends itself very well to being spiralized.

Favorite cooking methods: Roasted, spiralized, and sautéed.

Nutritional info: Kohlrabi contains a variety of nutrients but is very high in vitamin C. This water-soluble vitamin is necessary for the synthesis of collagen in the body and contributes to wound healing.

Selection: Choose kohlrabi that do not have any blemishes or dark spots on the skin. They should feel firm and heavy for their size.

Storage: Remove leaves and stalks, wrap in a damp paper towel, and store loosely in a sealed plastic bag. Kohlrabi bulbs should last for about 1 week in the produce drawer in the refrigerator.

Kohlrabi Noodles with Red Sauce and Kidney Beans

Serves 4 | Prep time: 10 minutes | Cook time: 15 minutes

Kohlrabi noodles hold up especially well in cooking and even resemble regular noodles. They capture the delicious flavor of marinara and the perfect texture of al dente spaghetti. The addition of kidney beans packs some more protein and fiber, which rounds out the dish nutritionally and makes it a quick vegetarian main dish for busy evenings.

- 2 tablespoons extra-virgin olive oil
- ½ yellow onion, diced
- 3 garlic cloves, minced
- 3 kohlrabi bulbs, trimmed and spiralized
- Homemade Tomato Sauce (page 158)
- ½ teaspoon dried oregano
- ½ teaspoon dried basil
- ⅛ teaspoon red pepper flakes (optional)
- Salt
- 1 (15-ounce) can red kidney beans, drained and rinsed

1. In a large skillet over medium heat, warm the olive oil. Add the onion and garlic and cook for 3 to 4 minutes, or until fragrant.
2. Add the kohlrabi noodles and cook, stirring frequently, for 5 to 7 minutes, or until softened.
3. Add the tomato sauce, oregano, basil, red pepper flakes (if using), and salt. Turn the heat to low and simmer for 5 to 7 minutes, or until warmed through.
4. Remove from the heat, mix in the kidney beans, and serve warm.

Notes: This meal tastes delicious with freshly grated vegan Parmesan cheese and a side of crunchy garlic bread.

Leeks and Scallions

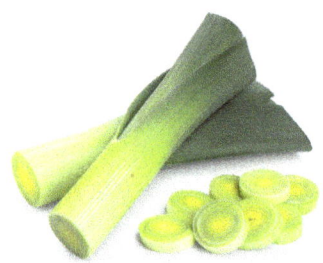

Season: Winter

Flavor profile: Leeks taste similar to their relatives: onions, shallots, scallions, and garlic. However, their flavor is milder and not as zesty compared to other types of onions. Raw leeks have a crunchy texture, while cooked leeks are tender and buttery. As with scallions, although all parts of a leek are edible, most recipes use only the white and light green parts.

Pairs with: Potatoes, garlic, thyme, rosemary, and white wine.

Varieties: Light green (less hardy leaves) and blue-green (hardier leaves).

Preparation: Cut off the bottoms and the dark green leaves on top, leaving just the white and light green parts of the stems. Cut in half, and rinse under cold running water. Use your fingers to gently open the layers as you rinse to ensure that you remove all of the dirt.

Favorite cooking methods: Roasted, braised, and sautéed.

Nutritional info: Leeks contain several of the same beneficial compounds as onions and garlic, including thiosulfinates that may help reduce blood pressure and boost heart health, among other benefits.

Selection: To get the most out of leeks, choose those that have long white and green stalks. The leaves should be firm, with a deep green color free of yellow spots.

Storage: You can keep leeks in a sealed bag or wrapped in plastic wrap in the produce drawer of the refrigerator. Use within 10 days.

Roasted Leeks

Serves 4 | Prep time: 10 minutes | Cook time: 20 minutes

Roasted leeks become wonderfully caramelized and have a mellow, almost sweet flavor. Add a little bit of salt and pepper to really showcase the mildly nutty flavor.

8 leeks, halved

1 tablespoon extra-virgin olive oil

Salt

Freshly ground black pepper

1. Preheat the oven to 400°F. Line a baking sheet with parchment paper.
2. Place the leeks on the prepared baking sheet, brush each side of the leeks with the olive oil, and position them cut-side down. Sprinkle with salt and pepper.
3. Roast for 10 minutes, flip the leeks over, and roast for another 10 minutes, or until slightly browned and tender.

Note: For more flavor, season the leeks with garlic powder before roasting.

Scallion Pancakes

Makes 4 pancakes | Prep time: 40 minutes | Cook time: 15 minutes

Savory scallion pancakes, made from a basic dough speckled with sliced scallions, are one of my favorite foods to order at Chinese restaurants. After years of enjoying them during dinners out, I was pleased to discover that they are incredibly easy to make at home.

FOR THE PANCAKES

- 2 cups all-purpose flour, plus more for rolling out the dough
- ½ teaspoon salt
- ½ teaspoon garlic powder
- ¾ cup just boiling water, plus more as needed
- ¼ cup canola oil, plus more for cooking
- 3 scallions, thinly sliced

FOR THE DIPPING SAUCE

- 2 tablespoons soy sauce
- 1 scallion, thinly sliced
- 1 tablespoon rice vinegar
- 1 teaspoon sesame oil
- 1 teaspoon maple syrup

1. **To make the pancakes:** In a large bowl, mix together the flour, salt, and garlic powder. Pour in the hot water and stir until the dough comes together. Using your hands, knead the dough for 2 minutes. If it's not sticking together, add 1 to 2 more tablespoons of hot water. The dough should be moist but not overly sticky. Shape the dough into a ball and cover the bowl with plastic wrap. Let it sit for 20 minutes.

2. Sprinkle a clean, dry work surface with flour. Cut the dough into 4 pieces and shape them into small balls. Using a rolling pin, roll out each dough ball into an 8-inch circle. Brush the surface of each circle with a thin layer of oil, and sprinkle about a quarter of the scallions over the surface of each circle.

3. Roll up one circle to make a log. Then take the right side of the log and curl it toward the center. The dough should look like a snail's shell at this point. Flatten the dough with your hand, then roll it out again into a thin circle. Repeat for the other dough circles.

4. In a skillet over medium heat, warm a small amount of canola oil or cooking spray. Cook each pancake for 2 to 3 minutes on each side, or until golden brown. Add more oil to the skillet in between pancakes as needed.

5. **To make the dipping sauce:** In a small bowl, whisk together the soy sauce, remaining scallion, vinegar, sesame oil, and maple syrup.

6. Serve the pancakes warm, cut into triangles, with the sauce on the side.

Lettuce

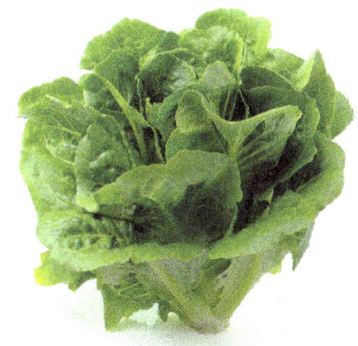

Season: Spring and Fall

Flavor profile: Fresh lettuce has a light, hydrating taste and crisp texture. Some varieties have a stronger flavor than others, but in general lettuce is mild and vegetal, with a high water content. Dressings and other toppings can completely transform the flavor profile of lettuce.

Pairs with: Vinaigrettes, creamy dressings, crunchy vegetables like carrots and radishes, and fresh and dried fruit.

Varieties: Romaine, butter, green or red leaf, and iceberg.

Preparation: Cut a head of lettuce in half, remove the core and ends, and separate the leaves. Wash under cold running water in a colander. Pat dry or use a salad spinner to remove excess water.

Favorite cooking methods: Raw in salads, stuffed, seared, and grilled.

Nutritional info: Since lettuce is mostly made of water, it's very low in calories, but it still packs several vitamins and minerals. Depending on the variety, lettuce may provide calcium, folate, phosphorus, and vitamins A, C, and K.

Selection: Choose heads of lettuce that have crisp leaves with no signs of wilting. The leaves should be intact, and iceberg lettuce in particular should be tightly packed.

Storage: Prepared and washed lettuce should be stored between paper towels in a plastic bag in the refrigerator for up to 1 week. Heads of lettuce can be loosely wrapped in paper towels and kept in the produce drawer for 10 days.

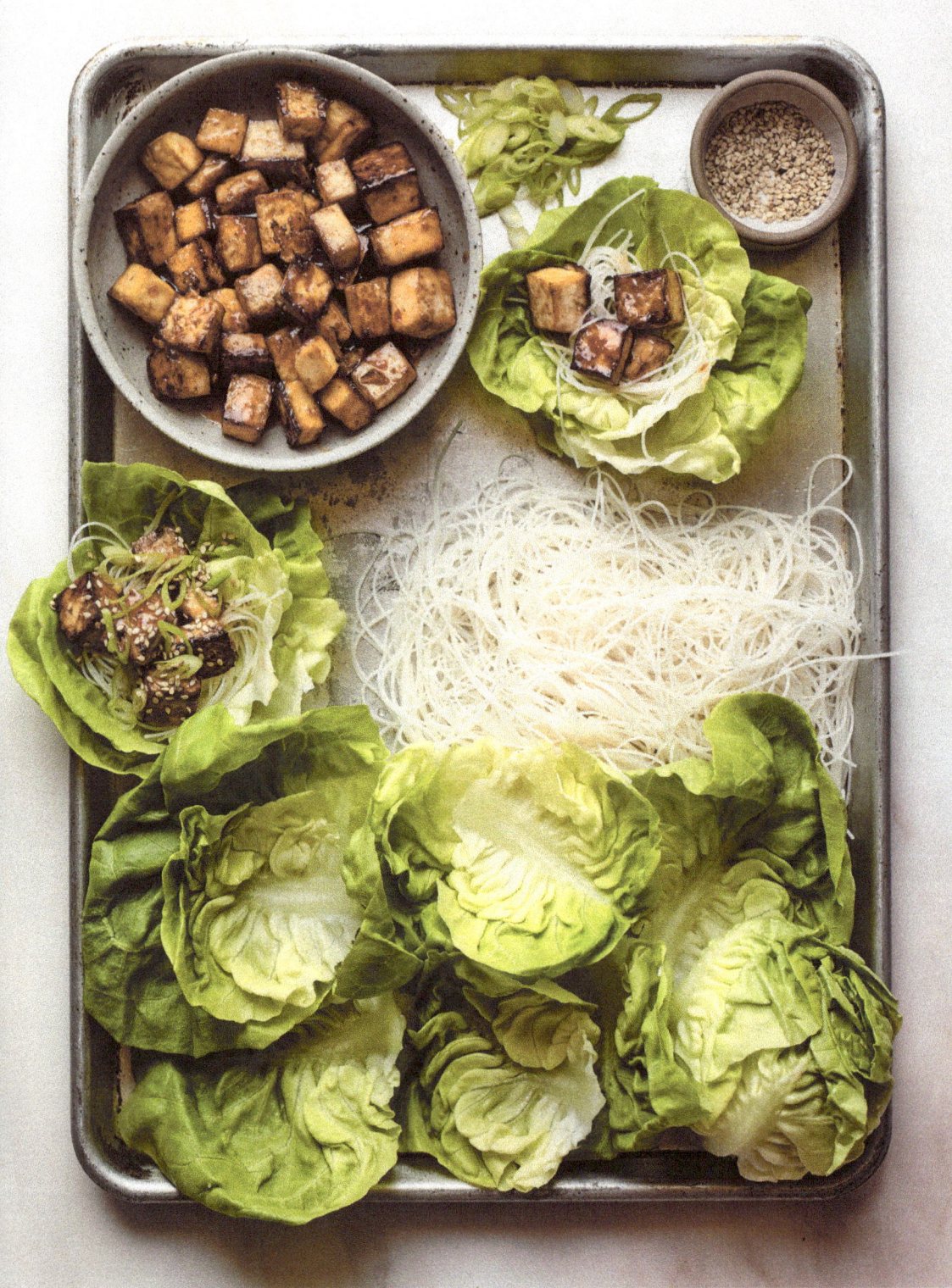

Vermicelli Lettuce Wraps

Serves 2 | Prep time: 25 minutes | Cook time: 40 minutes

A light and refreshing meal with a great crunchy texture, these wraps are perfect for a summer afternoon. This recipe is mostly about assembling—aside from cooking the tofu and vermicelli, all you have to do is chop some veggies and put it all together.

1 16-ounce block tofu

2 teaspoons coconut aminos

¼ cup sweet chili sauce

½ tablespoon hoisin sauce

1 teaspoon sriracha

1 teaspoon toasted sesame oil

1 package vermicelli noodles

2 heads Boston lettuce

1 scallion, chopped

1 teaspoon sesame seeds

1. Preheat the oven to 400°F. Line a baking sheet with parchment paper.
2. Drain the tofu and pat dry with paper towels. Place the tofu between two paper towels, then put something heavy, like a skillet, on top to help press out the excess water. Let sit for 15 minutes.
3. Cut the tofu into cubes, toss it with the coconut aminos, then spread it out evenly on the prepared baking sheet.
4. Bake for 35 minutes, flipping the tofu cubes halfway through.
5. In a small skillet over medium heat, combine the sweet chili sauce, hoisin sauce, sriracha, and toasted sesame oil.
6. Reduce the heat to low, add the baked tofu cubes, and cook for 5 minutes. Toss until evenly coated, then remove from the heat.
7. Cook the vermicelli noodles according to the package instructions.
8. To assemble the wraps, use 1 or 2 leaves of lettuce for each wrap. Layer the noodles and tofu, sprinkling the scallion and sesame seeds on top.

Grilled Romaine Lettuce

Serves 4 | Prep time: 5 minutes | Cook time: 5 minutes

Throw romaine lettuce on the grill for a delicious char. Use the lettuce in salads or as a delicious wrap, filled with tofu or tempeh.

4 romaine hearts

2 tablespoons extra-virgin olive oil

1 tablespoon apple cider vinegar

1 teaspoon garlic powder

¼ teaspoon salt

Freshly ground black pepper

1. Preheat the grill to medium-high.
2. Cut about 2 inches off of each head of romaine, and shave off the very bottom of the root, leaving it intact.
3. In a small bowl, whisk together the olive oil, vinegar, garlic powder, and salt. Season with pepper. Brush the mixture over all sides of the romaine.
4. Place the romaine directly on the grill or on a grilling mat and cook, turning the romaine with tongs so that it cooks evenly, for 1 to 2 minutes on each side, or until slightly charred.

Mushrooms

Season: Spring and Fall

Flavor profile: With a rich umami flavor and meaty texture, mushrooms are a common substitute for meat in vegetarian meals. Though they are technically a type of fungi, mushrooms are treated similarly to vegetables in the kitchen. Raw mushrooms have a mild, earthy taste, while cooked mushrooms soak up flavors like a sponge.

Pairs with: Garlic, onions, lemon, balsamic vinegar, soy sauce, sesame oil, paprika, rosemary, thyme, and oregano.

Varieties: Portobello, cremini, oyster, shiitake, white button, chanterelle, and porcini.

Preparation: Brush mushrooms with a damp paper towel to remove dirt. Use a knife to quarter or thinly slice, with or without the stems intact.

Favorite cooking methods: Sautéed, grilled, and stuffed.

Nutritional info: Mushrooms are a good source of water-soluble B vitamins, including niacin, riboflavin, thiamin, and pantothenic acid. B vitamins help the body metabolize food and extract energy from proteins, fats, and carbohydrates.

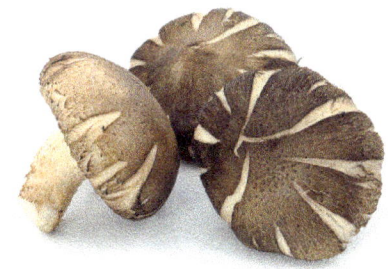

Selection: Mushrooms should be firm to the touch with a uniform color, and the caps should show no signs of shriveling. Avoid mushrooms that are slimy or appear dried out.

Storage: Place mushrooms in a brown paper bag, fold the top, and keep in the refrigerator. You can also keep them in their original packaging or a sealed container. Mushrooms last for at least 1 week.

Balsamic Roasted Mushrooms

Serves 4 | Prep time: 5 minutes | Cook time: 25 minutes

These balsamic roasted mushrooms are bursting with flavor. They are the perfect side dish to any meal and call for only a few simple ingredients.

2 tablespoons extra-virgin olive oil

1 tablespoon balsamic vinegar

1 tablespoon fresh thyme

1 teaspoon garlic powder

1 pound cremini mushrooms, quartered

Salt

1. Preheat the oven to 400°F. Line a baking sheet with parchment paper.
2. In a medium bowl, whisk together the olive oil, vinegar, thyme, and garlic powder. Add the mushrooms and mix until coated. Transfer the mushrooms to the prepared baking sheet and spread them out in a single layer. Season with salt.
3. Roast for 25 minutes, or until tender.

Mushroom Chips

Serves 4 | Prep time: 10 minutes | Cook time: 45 minutes

If you love the umami taste of mushrooms, this one is for you. The 'shrooms are thinly sliced and slow-roasted, making them highly concentrated with flavor. Mushroom chips are so potently delicious that you'll only need a handful to satisfy your snack craving. You can also enjoy them on salads.

2 Portobello mushrooms

2 tablespoons extra-virgin olive oil, plus more as needed

Salt

Freshly ground black pepper

1. Preheat the oven to 300°F. Line a baking sheet with parchment paper.
2. Carefully remove the stems of the mushrooms without tearing the caps. It's also helpful to peel the top layer of skin off of the caps so that they don't get stuck in the mandoline. Slice the mushrooms with a mandoline or use a sharp knife to cut them into ⅛-inch slices.
3. Arrange the sliced mushrooms in a single layer on the prepared baking sheet, making sure they don't overlap. Brush each side with a small amount of olive oil. Season with salt and pepper.
4. Bake for 45 to 50 minutes, or until the mushrooms are completely dry and crispy and have a dark color. Let them cool for a few minutes before eating.

Notes: Make sure the chips are crispy before taking them out of the oven, because they will not crisp up like other veggie chips at room temperature. Store in an airtight container at room temperature for up to 1 week.

Mushroom and Lentil Gravy

Serves 4 | Prep time: 5 minutes | Cook time: 25 minutes

Savory mushroom gravy is the ultimate comfort food, and the addition of lentils makes it a suitable source of protein to serve over roasted or mashed vegetables. You can thicken it with cornstarch to mimic traditional gravy or skip that step to serve it like a stew. I like to make this recipe for a cozy meal on a cold evening.

- 1 tablespoon extra-virgin olive oil
- 8 ounces cremini mushrooms, chopped
- 1 small yellow onion, diced
- ½ teaspoon dried thyme
- ½ teaspoon dried rosemary
- ½ cup green lentils
- 2 cups vegetable broth
- Salt
- 1 tablespoon cornstarch whisked together with 2 tablespoons water (optional)

1. In a large saucepan over medium heat, warm the olive oil. Add the mushrooms and onion and cook for 5 to 7 minutes, or until tender.
2. Add the thyme, rosemary, lentils, and broth and stir to combine. Season with salt. Raise the heat to medium-high and bring to a boil. Lower the heat to medium-low and simmer for 12 to 15 minutes, or until the lentils are tender.
3. If you want to thicken the gravy, add the cornstarch mixture to the gravy and cook, stirring constantly, until the gravy begins to thicken. Remove from the heat and serve warm.

Notes: Store leftovers in an airtight container in the refrigerator for up to 4 days. Reheat in a saucepan over medium-low heat, stirring frequently to prevent scorching.

Portobello Burgers

Serves 4 | Prep time: 5 minutes | Cook time: 20 minutes

The beauty of vegan portobello mushroom burgers is that you can have a vegan burger without having to make a patty. Portobello mushrooms are "meaty," and the texture holds up amazingly in a burger. Pair with your favorite burger toppings and fries for a delicious vegan replacement.

⅓ cup extra-virgin olive oil

1 teaspoon garlic powder

½ teaspoon mustard powder

1 tablespoon vegan Worcestershire sauce or low-sodium soy sauce

Dash cayenne pepper

4 large portobello mushrooms, stems and gills removed

Salt

Freshly ground black pepper

1. Preheat the oven to 375°F.
2. In a medium bowl, whisk together the olive oil, garlic powder, mustard powder, Worcestershire sauce, and cayenne.
3. Dip the mushroom caps in the mixture and place them stem-side down on a baking sheet. Sprinkle with salt and pepper. Bake for 20 minutes, or until softened.
4. Add your desired toppings and serve.

Okra

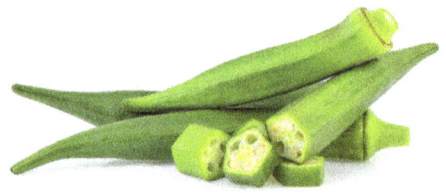

Season: Summer

Flavor profile: Okra can have a soft or crunchy texture depending on how it's cooked. The flavor is very mild.

Pairs with: Okra works best in sauces or with other vegetables in curries or stir-fries.

Varieties: Clemson spineless, burgundy, jambalaya, and heritage.

Preparation: Wash and slice your first, then let it dry. You can boil okra in slightly salted water or cook it dry over medium heat. To prevent your okra from getting slimy, soak the slices in 1 quart of water with 1 cup of vinegar for 1 hour. Always let it dry completely before cooking.

Favorite cooking methods: Sautéed, fried, and baked.

Nutritional info: Okra is loaded with antioxidants and polyphenols, which decrease your risk of heart problems and stroke. It contains magnesium, folate, vitamin A, vitamin C, vitamin K and vitamin B_6.

Selection: Select okra that is firm and bright in color.

Storage: Store okra in your refrigerator.

Okra Curry

Serves 2 | Prep time: 15 minutes | Cook time: 20 minutes

You can easily pick up the ingredients you need for this tasty aromatic curry at any grocery store. In fact, you might have a lot of the ingredients already in your kitchen right now. Don't be intimated by the spices—they really bring out the authentic flavor. Pair this curry with basmati rice for a hearty meal.

1 cup okra

2 tablespoons coconut oil

1 small yellow onion, diced

3 garlic cloves, minced

1 teaspoon grated fresh ginger

½ teaspoon dried thyme

1 small tomato, chopped

2 tablespoons curry powder

¼ teaspoon ground allspice

½ Scotch bonnet pepper

1 cup canned coconut milk

¼ cup vegetable broth

Salt

1. Place the okra in a colander and rinse under cold water. Cut off the stems and set aside.
2. In a large saucepan, warm the coconut oil over medium heat. Add the onion, garlic, ginger, and thyme and cook, stirring, for about 2 minutes, or until the onion is soft.
3. Stir in the tomato and cook for 1 minute.
4. Add the curry powder, allspice, and Scotch bonnet pepper and stir. Cook for 1 minute.
5. Add the okra and stir to coat it with the seasonings. Stir in the coconut milk, broth, and salt to taste. Bring the curry to a boil. Cook for 10 minutes, or until the okra is tender. Serve with rice.

Onions and Shallots

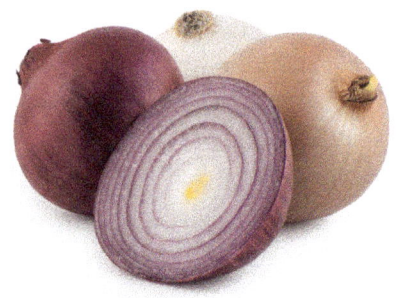

Season: Spring, Fall, and Winter

Flavor profile: Depending on the type, the taste of onions ranges from strong and zesty to sweet and mild. They are one of the most versatile and widely used foods, adding base flavor to soups, stir-fries, sauces, and more.

Pairs with: Garlic, carrots, celery, olive oil, black pepper, thyme, and balsamic vinegar.

Varieties: Yellow, sweet, white, red, shallots, and cipolline (which are dry onions harvested once they're mature, providing a juicy, sweet flavor).

Preparation: Trim the top, and peel off the papery skin with your fingers. To dice an onion, cut it in half, then make vertical cuts from the end to the top (½ inch apart), followed by perpendicular cuts across each half. Remove and discard the ends after dicing.

Favorite cooking methods: Sautéed, roasted, caramelized, and pickled.

Nutritional info: Onions provide vitamin C, potassium, and several antioxidant compounds. They are also rich in prebiotic fibers called fructans that feed gut bacteria.

Selection: Fresh onions are firm and heavy, with dry skins and tight necks. Old or rotten onions feel soft or mushy.

Storage: Onions can be stored for up to 4 weeks in a cool, dry spot in the kitchen.

Okra Curry

Serves 2 | Prep time: 15 minutes | Cook time: 20 minutes

You can easily pick up the ingredients you need for this tasty aromatic curry at any grocery store. In fact, you might have a lot of the ingredients already in your kitchen right now. Don't be intimated by the spices—they really bring out the authentic flavor. Pair this curry with basmati rice for a hearty meal.

1 cup okra

2 tablespoons coconut oil

1 small yellow onion, diced

3 garlic cloves, minced

1 teaspoon grated fresh ginger

½ teaspoon dried thyme

1 small tomato, chopped

2 tablespoons curry powder

¼ teaspoon ground allspice

½ Scotch bonnet pepper

1 cup canned coconut milk

¼ cup vegetable broth

Salt

1. Place the okra in a colander and rinse under cold water. Cut off the stems and set aside.
2. In a large saucepan, warm the coconut oil over medium heat. Add the onion, garlic, ginger, and thyme and cook, stirring, for about 2 minutes, or until the onion is soft.
3. Stir in the tomato and cook for 1 minute.
4. Add the curry powder, allspice, and Scotch bonnet pepper and stir. Cook for 1 minute.
5. Add the okra and stir to coat it with the seasonings. Stir in the coconut milk, broth, and salt to taste. Bring the curry to a boil. Cook for 10 minutes, or until the okra is tender. Serve with rice.

Onions and Shallots

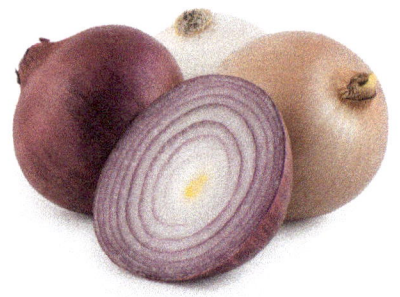

Season: Spring, Fall, and Winter

Flavor profile: Depending on the type, the taste of onions ranges from strong and zesty to sweet and mild. They are one of the most versatile and widely used foods, adding base flavor to soups, stir-fries, sauces, and more.

Pairs with: Garlic, carrots, celery, olive oil, black pepper, thyme, and balsamic vinegar.

Varieties: Yellow, sweet, white, red, shallots, and cipolline (which are dry onions harvested once they're mature, providing a juicy, sweet flavor).

Preparation: Trim the top, and peel off the papery skin with your fingers. To dice an onion, cut it in half, then make vertical cuts from the end to the top (½ inch apart), followed by perpendicular cuts across each half. Remove and discard the ends after dicing.

Favorite cooking methods: Sautéed, roasted, caramelized, and pickled.

Nutritional info: Onions provide vitamin C, potassium, and several antioxidant compounds. They are also rich in prebiotic fibers called fructans that feed gut bacteria.

Selection: Fresh onions are firm and heavy, with dry skins and tight necks. Old or rotten onions feel soft or mushy.

Storage: Onions can be stored for up to 4 weeks in a cool, dry spot in the kitchen.

Make-Ahead Caramelized Onions

Serves 4 | Prep time: 5 minutes | Cook time: 45 minutes

Caramelized onions are such a staple and add mouthwatering flavor to almost any dish. From quiches to pizzas, burgers, and sandwiches, this is one ingredient that will take your cooking up to a new level.

- 2 tablespoons extra-virgin olive oil
- 2 onions, thinly sliced
- ½ teaspoon salt

In a large skillet over medium heat, warm the olive oil. Add the onions and salt, and stir until evenly coated. Lower the heat to medium-low and cook, stirring every few minutes, for 40 to 50 minutes, or until the onions are caramelized and tender. Pour in a splash of water as needed to deglaze the pan and scrape up the brown bits if the onions start to stick.

Notes: Store the onions in an airtight container in the refrigerator for up to 1 week and add to recipes as desired. You can also freeze them in a zip-top plastic bag or in smaller portions in an ice cube tray covered with a plastic bag for up to 3 months.

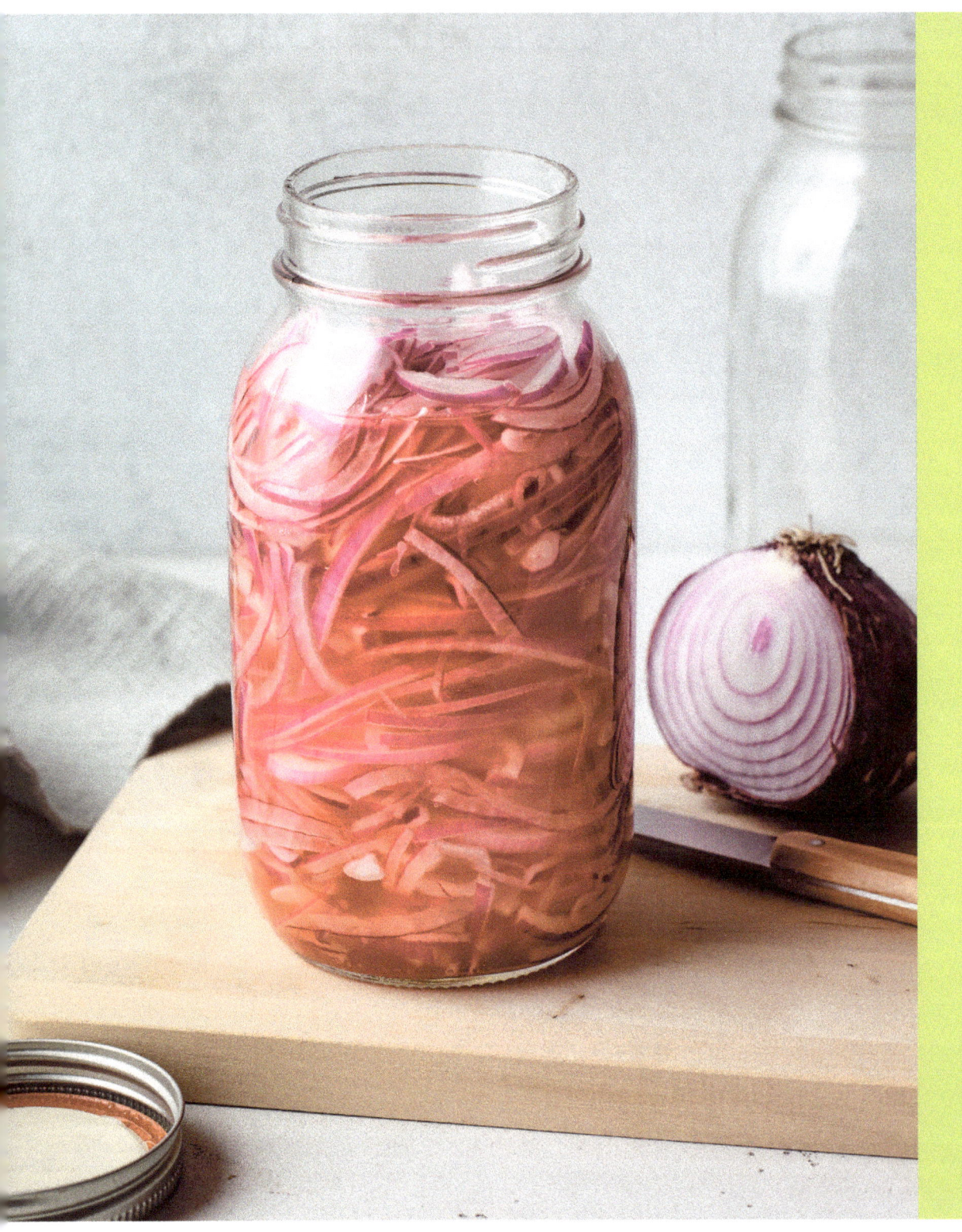

Quick Pickled Red Onions

Makes 2 (8-ounce) jars | Prep time: 10 minutes, plus 30 minutes to pickle | Cook time: 5 minutes

Pickled red onions are my favorite vegetable-based condiment. They add a yummy crunch and burst of sweet, tangy flavor to tacos, sandwiches, nachos, avocado toast, and more. They disappear pretty quickly in our household. Luckily, this recipe takes almost no time to prepare and uses basic pantry ingredients, so I can whip up a batch every week if needed.

1 red onion, thinly sliced
½ cup apple cider vinegar
1 tablespoon granulated sugar
1 teaspoon salt
½ cup water

1. Divide the onions equally between two 8-ounce jars. (You can also use one 16-ounce jar instead.)
2. In a small saucepan over medium heat, combine the vinegar, sugar, salt, and water. Bring to a simmer, stirring until the sugar dissolves. Remove from the heat and pour the brine equally over the onions.
3. Seal the jars and let the onions sit for 30 minutes at room temperature. Transfer the jars to the refrigerator and use within 3 weeks.

Notes: You can substitute white wine vinegar or red wine vinegar for the apple cider vinegar. For some added flavor, mix in 2 teaspoons of whole peppercorns, fennel seeds, or caraway seeds. Avocado Toast with Quick Pickled Red Onions (page 23) is a tasty way to use these onions.

French Lentil and Shallot Soup

Serves 4 to 6 | Prep time: 10 minutes | Cook time: 45 minutes

This mouthwatering dish is reminiscent of traditional French onion soup, but with fully vegetarian ingredients and a shorter cook time. Sliced shallots are quickly caramelized before they simmer with lentils in a rich vegetable broth spiked with Worcestershire sauce. Be sure to serve this soup with a toasted French baguette to soak up every last drop.

4 tablespoons extra-virgin olive oil

6 shallots, thinly sliced

2 garlic cloves, minced

1 teaspoon dried thyme

2 tablespoons all-purpose flour

6 cups vegetable broth

1 tablespoon vegan Worcestershire sauce

2 bay leaves

1 cup French lentils, sorted and rinsed

1. In a large stockpot over medium heat, warm the olive oil. Add the shallots and cook for 10 to 15 minutes, or until they are tender and slightly caramelized.
2. Add the garlic, thyme, and flour and cook for another 3 to 4 minutes.
3. Raise the heat to medium-high. Add the broth, Worcestershire sauce, bay leaves, and lentils and bring to a boil. Lower the heat to medium-low, cover, and simmer for 20 to 25 minutes, or until the lentils are tender. Remove and discard the bay leaves before serving.

Notes: For additional flavor, add ½ cup of white wine and 1 tablespoon of balsamic vinegar when you add the broth. Use gluten-free all-purpose flour to make this dish gluten-free.

Parsnips

Season: Fall and Winter

Flavor profile: Although they look like pale carrots, parsnips have a distinct flavor that's sweet and nutty with hints of licorice brought out by roasting. They're also starchier than carrots and have a creamy consistency when cooked.

Pairs with: Olive oil, cinnamon, nutmeg, raisins, maple syrup, apples, sage, garlic, pears, carrots, and potatoes.

Varieties: Several that range in color from off-white to light yellow.

Preparation: Scrub clean with a vegetable brush and remove the skin with a swivel peeler if desired. Slice or dice with a sharp knife.

Favorite cooking methods: Roasted, shaved, shredded, and mashed.

Nutritional info: Parsnips provide several micronutrients and are a good source of vitamin C, which helps protect cells from free radical damage associated with disease development.

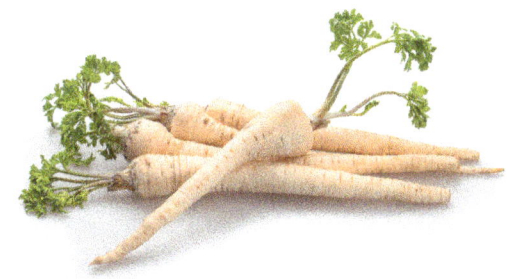

Selection: Look for parsnips that are firm and unblemished. They should not feel soft or appear shriveled.

Storage: Keep parsnips in a sealed plastic bag in the crisper drawer. If the greens are attached, cut them off 1 inch from the roots before storing. They can be stored for up to 2 weeks.

Thyme Roasted Parsnip Coins

Serves 4 | Prep time: 5 minutes | Cook time: 25 minutes

Roasted parsnips are simple to make and incredibly delicious as a vegetable side to any dinner. They have a natural sweetness that caramelizes in the oven for a delicious flavor.

6 parsnips, cut into ½-inch coins

2 tablespoons extra-virgin olive oil

1 teaspoon dried thyme, or 1 tablespoon fresh thyme

Salt

1. Preheat the oven to 400°F. Line a baking sheet with parchment paper.
2. In a large bowl, toss the parsnips with the olive oil and thyme until evenly coated. Arrange the parsnip coins in a single layer on the baking sheet and season with salt.
3. Roast, stirring the parsnips halfway through, for 25 to 35 minutes, or until tender and browned.

Parsnip and Apple Soup

Serves 4 to 6 | Prep time: 10 minutes | Cook time: 40 minutes

As soon as the leaves begin to change colors, signifying the start of apple and root vegetable season, I make a batch of this flavorful soup. It's the kind of dish that warms you from the inside out, and every spoonful oozes coziness. Serve it with a large slice of crunchy bread on the side.

- 2 tablespoons extra-virgin olive oil
- 2 shallots, diced
- 1 tablespoon fresh thyme
- 5 parsnips, peeled and cut into ½-inch rounds
- 3 apples, cored and diced
- Salt
- 4 cups vegetable broth

1. In a large stockpot over medium-high heat, warm the olive oil. Add the shallots and cook for 3 to 5 minutes, or until softened.
2. Add the thyme, parsnips, and apples, and cook for another 5 to 7 minutes. Season with salt.
3. Add the broth, stir to combine, and bring to a boil. Lower the heat to medium-low and cook for 20 to 25 minutes, or until the parsnips are fork-tender.
4. Remove the soup from the heat and puree with an immersion blender until smooth. Serve warm.

Notes: My favorite types of apples to use in this recipe include Pink Lady and Honeycrisp or a combination of these with a Granny Smith apple. To blend the soup safely in a regular blender, fill it halfway and puree the soup in batches. Leave a corner of the lid cracked, or remove the top of the blender and cover it with a folded dish towel to let steam escape as you blend. Be careful not to get burned by the steam.

Peas and Peapods

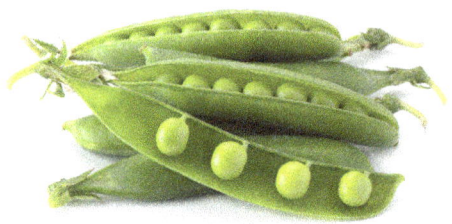

Season: Spring

Flavor profile: Fresh green peas are deliciously sweet, with earthy undertones and a starchy texture. Snow and sugar snap peas are typically eaten with their pods, which are crisp and fibrous.

Pairs with: Garlic, shallots, carrots, asparagus, dill, mint, lemon, soy sauce, sesame oil, and red pepper.

Varieties: Green (garden), snow, and sugar snap.

Preparation: Trim pods before cooking or eating raw. To shell peas, use a knife or your fingers to pop open the pods and pluck out the peas.

Favorite cooking methods: Raw, stir-fried, and roasted.

Nutritional info: Peas contain fiber, folate, iron, manganese, and vitamin C. They are also higher in protein than most other vegetables.

Selection: Choose peapods that are bright green and free from bruises or discoloration. Loose peas should be plump and firm, without any evidence of shriveling.

Storage: Keep peapods in a sealed plastic bag or container in the refrigerator for up to 5 days. Shelled peas can be stored the same way if you plan to use them within a couple of days. Otherwise, blanch shelled peas for 2 minutes in boiling water, submerge them in ice water to cool, drain, and freeze in a plastic bag for up to 3 months.

Sautéed Green Peas with Dill

Serves 4 | Prep time: 5 minutes | Cook time: 10 minutes

Peas are sometimes thought of as a mushy mess on a cafeteria tray, but when they're properly prepared, they add a crisp pop of flavor that's impossible to resist. With this recipe, you'll see what I mean in just 15 minutes. Freshly shaved vegan Parmesan cheese and a touch of fresh dill highlight the vegetal taste of fresh peas to make a perfect side dish.

1 tablespoon extra-virgin olive oil

3 garlic cloves, minced

2 cups green peas

1 tablespoon chopped fresh dill

Freshly ground black pepper

Freshly shaved vegan Parmesan cheese, for serving

1. In a large skillet over medium heat, warm the olive oil. Add the garlic and cook for about 2 minutes, or until fragrant.
2. Add the peas and dill and season with pepper. Cook for 5 to 7 minutes, or until the peas are tender.
3. Remove from the heat and serve topped with freshly shaved cheese.

Notes: You can use fresh or frozen peas for this recipe. Frozen peas do not need to be thawed before being added to the skillet.

Snap Pea and Barley Salad with Shallot Dijon Vinaigrette

Serves 4 to 6 | Prep time: 10 minutes

This healthy grain-based salad may look overly simple, but it has a complex flavor profile thanks to the shallot dressing and the combination of textures. Sugar snap peas provide a refreshing crispness that offsets the chewy consistency of barley and the buttery mouthfeel of chickpeas. With so much to offer, this recipe is bound to become your go-to weekday lunch.

FOR THE VINAIGRETTE

¼ cup extra-virgin olive oil
⅛ cup apple cider vinegar
1½ teaspoons maple syrup
½ teaspoon Dijon mustard
1 large shallot, finely chopped
¾ teaspoon Himalayan salt
¼ teaspoon freshly ground black pepper
Pinch crushed red pepper flakes

FOR THE SALAD

2 cups cooked pearl barley
1 pound sugar snap peas, trimmed and halved
1 (15-ounce) can chickpeas, drained and rinsed

TO MAKE THE VINAIGRETTE

1. In a mason jar or other glass jar with a tight-fitting lid, combine the olive oil, vinegar, maple syrup, mustard, shallot, salt, black pepper, and red pepper flakes. Shake vigorously until well mixed.

TO MAKE THE SALAD

2. In a large bowl, mix together the barley, snap peas, and chickpeas.
3. Add the vinaigrette and toss until evenly coated. Serve immediately or refrigerate to chill.

Notes: Cook the barley according to the package instructions. Trader Joe's and other stores offer quick-cooking varieties that can save you time. You can prep both the barley and the dressing in advance and put the salad together when you're ready to eat. Leftovers can be stored in an airtight container in the refrigerator for up to 5 days.

Peppers

Season: Summer

Flavor profile: Ranging from sweet and mild to spicy and hot, the flavor profile of peppers largely depends on the type. Pepper seeds, especially from jalapeño or serrano peppers, contribute additional heat if they're not removed. In terms of texture, peppers have crunchy, juicy flesh.

Pairs with: Fresh herbs, lime, red wine vinegar, hummus, garlic, black beans, and pinto beans.

Varieties: Green, red, yellow, and orange bell peppers, jalapeños, serranos, chiles, and habaneros.

Preparation: Cut off the stem, cut the pepper in half, and remove the seeds with a spoon, a knife, or your hands (be careful not to touch your face after cutting spicy peppers). Bell peppers can be diced or cut into strips, but spicy peppers should be more finely minced.

Favorite cooking methods: Raw, roasted, and sautéed.

Nutritional info: All types of peppers contain several vitamins and minerals, including high amounts of vitamin C. The compound in hot peppers that makes them spicy, known as capsaicin, may help improve digestion and relieve pain.

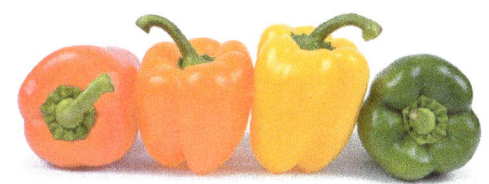

Selection: Fresh peppers have firm, glossy skin and feel heavy for their size. They should have no brown or black spots.

Storage: Keep peppers dry to prevent rotting. Place them in a sealed plastic bag or wrap tightly with plastic wrap, and store in the produce drawer of the refrigerator for up to 5 days.

Roasted Red Peppers

Serves 4 to 6 | Prep time: 10 minutes | Cook time: 20 minutes

With only one main ingredient, this recipe is incredibly simple but bursting with flavor. Roasting peppers adds a vibrant and complex flavor.

4 red bell peppers, seeded and cut in half

¼ cup extra-virgin olive oil

3 garlic cloves, minced

Salt

Freshly ground black pepper

1. Preheat the oven to 450°F. Line a baking sheet with aluminum foil.
2. Arrange the peppers cut-side down in a single layer on the prepared baking sheet. Roast for 20 to 25 minutes, or until wilted and charred. Let cool for a few minutes.
3. Rinse each pepper under cold water and, using your fingers, peel off the skin. Transfer the peeled peppers to a cutting board and cut into thin slices.
4. Place the peppers in a glass jar with a lid or in an airtight container. Add the olive oil and garlic, season with salt and pepper, and toss to combine.

Notes: The peppers will keep in the refrigerator for up to 2 weeks. You can also freeze them in zip-top plastic bags for up to 3 months.

Fresh Bell Pepper and Herb Salad

Serves 4 | Prep time: 15 minutes

If you have a vegetable garden with pepper plants and herbs during the warm months, this recipe is a wonderful way to enjoy the fruits of your labor. Crunchy, refreshing bell peppers, combined with a variety of herbs, make for an irresistibly fresh salad that captures the essence of the summer harvest. I love to use a mix of red, orange, and yellow bell peppers to make this dish as colorful as possible.

FOR THE SALAD

2 large bell peppers, seeded and cut into rings

1 small shallot, cut into rings

¼ cup red wine vinegar

Salt

FOR THE DRESSING

1 tablespoon extra-virgin olive oil

1 tablespoon chopped fresh mint

1 tablespoon chopped fresh basil

1 tablespoon chopped fresh parsley

1 tablespoon chopped fresh dill

TO MAKE THE SALAD

1. In a large bowl, toss the sliced bell peppers and shallots in the vinegar. Sprinkle with salt. Let the salad sit for about 10 minutes so that the vinegar softens the peppers, if desired.

TO MAKE THE DRESSING

2. In a small bowl, mix together the olive oil, mint, basil, parsley, and dill.

3. Add the dressing to the salad and toss until evenly coated.

Notes: This salad tastes even better when it sits in the refrigerator for a couple of hours to let the flavors meld together. You can store it in an airtight container in the refrigerator for up to 1 day in advance for maximum flavor.

Stuffed Pepper Soup

Serves 4 to 6 | Prep time: 5 minutes | Cook time: 40 minutes

For the same delicious flavors of stuffed peppers without the hassle of eating them with a fork and knife, I give you stuffed pepper soup. This low-maintenance dish calls for mostly pantry staples plus fresh bell peppers. With plenty of vegetables, brown rice, and pinto beans, it's a nutritious and balanced meal in one bowl.

- 1 tablespoon extra-virgin olive oil
- 1 yellow onion, diced
- 4 garlic cloves, minced
- ½ teaspoon salt, plus more as needed
- 2 bell peppers, diced
- 1 (14-ounce) can fire-roasted diced tomatoes
- ½ teaspoon dried oregano
- ½ teaspoon dried thyme
- 1 cup short-grain brown rice
- 4 cups vegetable broth
- 1 (15-ounce) can pinto beans, drained and rinsed

1. In a large pot over medium heat, warm the olive oil. Add the onion, garlic, and salt, and cook for 3 to 4 minutes, or until fragrant.
2. Add the bell peppers, tomatoes, oregano, and thyme, and cook for another 3 to 4 minutes.
3. Add the rice and broth, stir, and bring to a boil. Lower the heat to medium-low and simmer, stirring occasionally, for about 30 minutes, or until the rice is tender.
4. Stir in the pinto beans, taste, and add more salt as needed. Ladle into bowls and serve.

Notes: If you don't eat all of the soup right away, the rice will continue to absorb the liquid. Add some more broth or water when reheating. Leftovers can be stored in an airtight container in the refrigerator for up to 4 days.

Potatoes

Season: Fall and Winter

Flavor profile: Plain potatoes have an earthy taste that's especially concentrated in the skin, and a starchy flesh that becomes tender when cooked. However, potatoes are more commonly enjoyed mashed, fried, or stuffed, with salt and other fixings that have made them an iconic comfort food.

Pairs with: Salt, leeks, shallots, onions, garlic, broccoli, rosemary, chives, chili powder, and paprika.

Varieties: Russet, red, Yukon gold, fingerling, purple, new, and several other varieties.

Preparation: Scrub clean with a vegetable brush. Keep potatoes whole, cut into slices with a mandoline for chips, or dice into pieces. Remove the skin with a swivel peeler if desired.

Favorite cooking methods: Baked, made into chips and fries, and mashed.

Nutritional info: Due to their starch content, potatoes are high in carbohydrates and very filling. They are also an excellent source of potassium, a mineral that's necessary for blood pressure regulation.

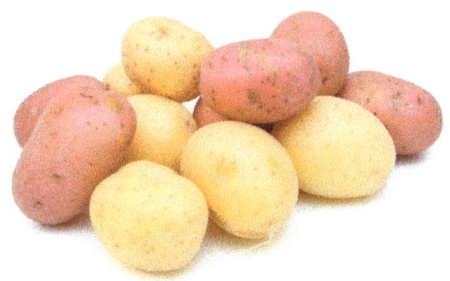

Selection: Look for potatoes that are firm to the touch, with no dark spots. Sprouts on the skin of potatoes are harmless but do indicate that they're older and should be removed before cooking. Avoid potatoes that have a green tinge, as they contain the toxic compound solanine.

Storage: Keep potatoes in a mesh or paper bag, basket, or cardboard box in a cool, dry, and dark place. They can last for at least a couple of weeks and sometimes longer.

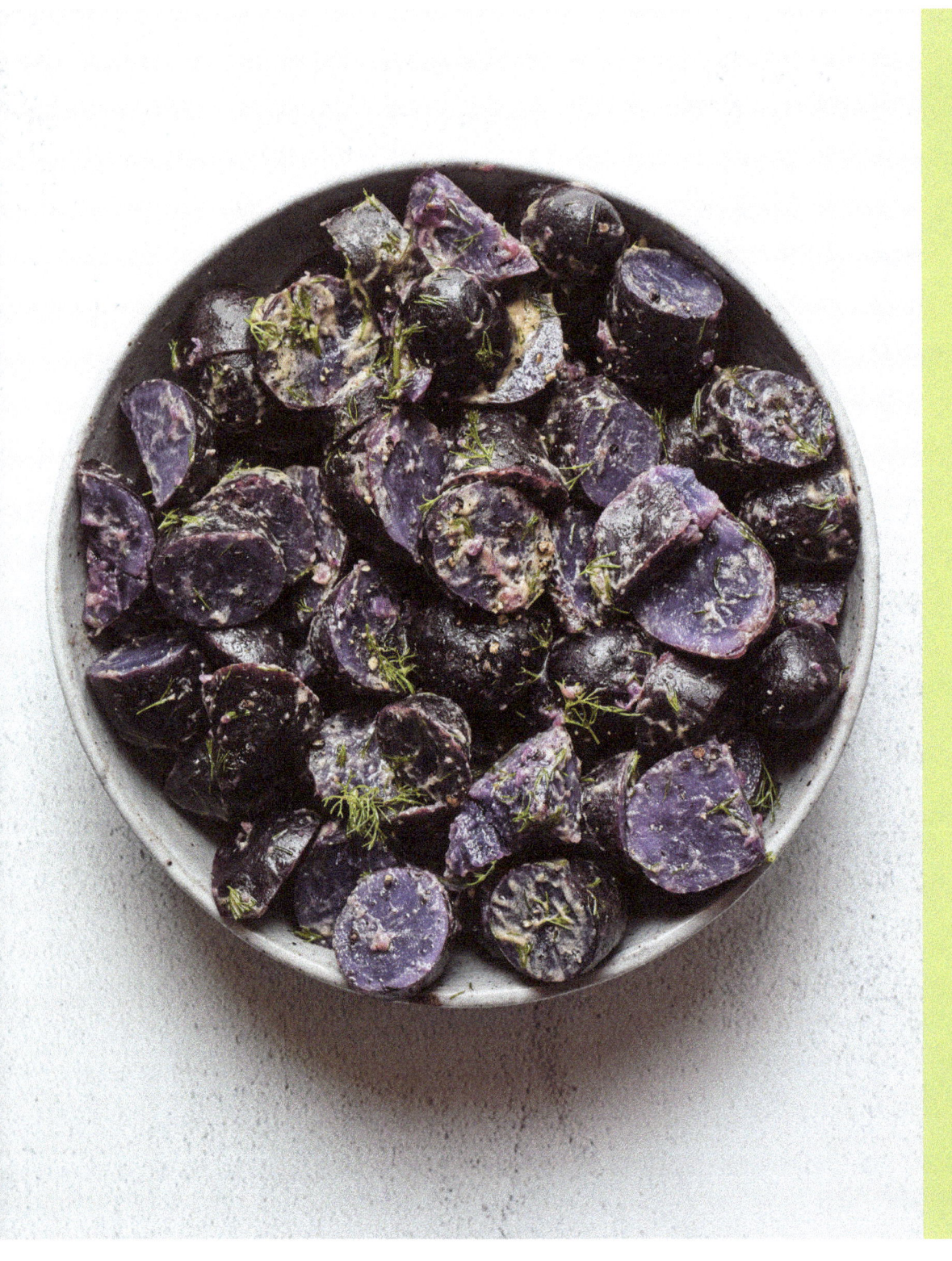

Olive Oil Purple Potato Salad

Serves 4 to 6 | Prep time: 10 minutes | Cook time: 10 minutes

The beautiful flesh of purple potatoes makes this recipe a real stunner, but it's more than just a pretty face. Purple potatoes get their color from anthocyanins, pigments that act as antioxidants in the body and may help improve vision and boost heart health. Plus, this dish swaps in olive oil for traditional mayonnaise, making it a lighter twist on classic potato salad. It's one of my go-to recipes for potlucks, cookouts, and holidays. If you're unable to find purple potatoes, you can easily substitute any other varieties you might have on hand.

2 pounds purple potatoes, cut into bite-size pieces

Salt

¼ cup extra-virgin olive oil

1 tablespoon Dijon mustard

1 tablespoon white wine vinegar

2 tablespoons chopped fresh dill

Freshly ground black pepper

1. Place the potatoes in a large pot, cover with water, add a few pinches of salt, and bring to a boil. Lower the heat to medium-low and cook for 6 to 8 minutes, or until the potatoes are fork-tender. Drain the potatoes and transfer to a large bowl.

2. In a small bowl, whisk together the olive oil, mustard, vinegar, and dill.

3. Add the olive oil mixture to the potatoes and toss until evenly coated. Season with salt and pepper.

Notes: Substitute the juice of ½ lemon for the white wine vinegar.

Paprika Baked Potato Chips

Serves 4 | Prep time: 10 minutes | Cook time: 20 minutes

Potato chips rank high on my list of favorite snacks, and I've been determined to figure out the best recipe for homemade chips over the past few years. Based on my experimentation, it's key to thinly slice the potatoes, using a high-starch variety like russets, and coat the chips with just enough oil before they go into the oven. Following those tips will yield a crunchy snack that most closely mimics store-bought chips.

3 teaspoons extra-virgin olive oil, divided

1 russet potato, thinly sliced with a mandoline

1 teaspoon smoked paprika

Salt

1. Preheat the oven to 400°F. Line two baking sheets with parchment paper. Brush the parchment paper with about 1 teaspoon of olive oil.

2. Brush the potato slices with the remaining 2 teaspoons of olive oil, coating each with a very thin layer of oil. Arrange them in a single layer on the baking sheets.

3. Bake the potatoes for 10 minutes, flip them over, rotate the pans, and bake for another 10 minutes. Some of the chips may cook faster than others, so keep an eye on them and take them off the sheets early if needed.

4. Once the edges of the chips are crispy, remove the baking sheet from the oven and let the chips cool for 5 minutes. Transfer to a bowl and toss with the paprika and salt to taste.

Notes: Using a mandoline is the best way to cut the potatoes into very thin slices for this recipe, but you can also use a sharp knife. These are best enjoyed right away, since they will lose their crispiness over time.

Scalloped Potatoes

Serves 4 Prep time: 20 minutes Cook time: 1 hour

Potatoes are the ultimate comfort food. The vegan ingredients in this dish give it the texture and flavor of the classic version, with the same dose of nostalgia. The coconut milk adds creaminess and a subtle sweetness that is delicious with the soft potatoes and sauce.

- 1 tablespoon extra-virgin olive oil
- 1 medium yellow onion, diced
- 2 (14-ounce) cans coconut milk
- 1 cup raw cashews, soaked overnight or boiled for 15 minutes and drained
- ½ teaspoon freshly ground black pepper
- 1 tablespoon Dijon mustard
- ½ cup nutritional yeast
- 1 teaspoon sea salt
- 1 teaspoon onion powder
- 1 teaspoon garlic powder
- 7 medium Yukon gold potatoes, peeled and thinly sliced
- Chopped chives, for garnish

1. Preheat the oven to 350°F.
2. In a small skillet over medium heat, warm the olive oil. Add the onion and sauté for 7 minutes.
3. In a high-speed blender, blend the onion, coconut milk, cashews, pepper, mustard, nutritional yeast, salt, onion powder, and garlic powder until very smooth. Set aside.
4. Layer half the potatoes in a 9-by-13-inch oven-safe dish. Pour half of the sauce over them, then layer on the rest of the potatoes. Spread the remaining sauce on top. Cover with aluminum foil and bake for 45 minutes, or until the potatoes are soft.
5. Remove the foil, then bake for a further 15 minutes. Allow to cool for 10 minutes, sprinkle with chopped chives, and serve.

Radishes

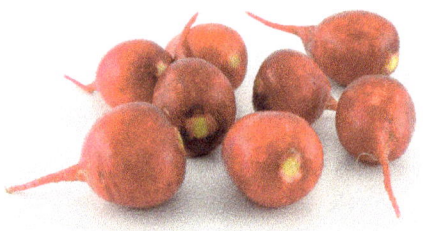

Season: Spring and Winter

Flavor profile: Raw radishes are peppery and slightly spicy, contributing a wonderful crunch and a zesty punch to dishes. Cooked radishes are tender and mellow. Radish leaves are also edible and can be used in pesto, stir-fries, and other dishes.

Pairs with: Dill, rosemary, mint, lemon, vinegars, sea salt, bread, and whole grains.

Varieties: Red, pink, purple, white, black, Daikon, and watermelon.

Preparation: Trim off the leaves and scrub the roots clean. Use whole, thinly slice with a mandoline, or chop into pieces.

Favorite cooking methods: Shaved or grated, roasted, and pickled.

Nutritional info: Radishes are rich in fiber and provide small amounts of potassium and vitamin C. They also contain compounds that have been shown to prevent cancer cell growth in test tube studies.

Selection: Choose radishes that feel firm, have smooth skin, and are bright in color. If their leaves are attached, they should be free of yellow spots and not wilting.

Storage: Use your hands to pluck the radishes from their greens. Wrap the loose radishes in a damp paper towel and keep in a sealed plastic bag for up to 2 weeks. Store radishes that have already been cut in an airtight container covered with water to keep them crispy.

Tarragon Roasted Radishes

Serves 4 | Prep time: 5 minutes | Cook time: 25 minutes

Radishes are typically served in soup or salad, but this roasted version with the subtle licorice flavor from the tarragon will change what you think of them forever.

2 bunches radishes, trimmed

1 tablespoon extra-virgin olive oil

2 tablespoons chopped fresh tarragon

Salt

Freshly ground black pepper

1. Preheat the oven to 400°F. Line a baking sheet with parchment paper.
2. Place the radishes on the prepared baking sheet and toss with the olive oil and tarragon. Arrange them in a single layer on the baking sheet and sprinkle with salt and pepper.
3. Bake for 25 to 30 minutes, or until the radishes are fork-tender.

Radish Chips

Serves 4 | Prep time: 5 minutes | Cook time: 15 minutes

These simple veggie chips make a great snack for after school or work. They taste delicious with just a sprinkle of salt and pepper, and you can have them on the table in only 20 minutes. If there are any left after you satisfy your snack attack (doubtful), throw them on salads or dip in hummus.

3 bunches radishes, thinly sliced

1 tablespoon extra-virgin olive oil

Salt

Freshly ground black pepper

1. Preheat the oven to 400°F. Line two baking sheets with parchment paper.
2. In a large bowl, toss the radishes in the olive oil until they are very lightly coated. Arrange them in a single layer on the baking sheets without overlapping.
3. Bake for 12 to 15 minutes, until the radishes are crispy and wrinkled. Check on them frequently, starting at 10 minutes, to make sure they don't burn.
4. Let the radishes cool for a couple of minutes. Season with salt and pepper, and enjoy.

Notes: A mandoline works best for cutting the radishes into thin slices, but you can also use a sharp knife. For a spicy kick, sprinkle the chips with a pinch of cayenne pepper before eating.

Rhubarb

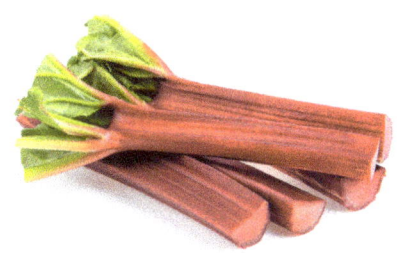

Season: Spring

Flavor profile: Although it may look like a pink version of celery, rhubarb has a different and very distinct taste. Raw rhubarb is tart and sour, but cooked rhubarb is sweeter and commonly used in desserts. Recipes with rhubarb only call for the stalks, since the leaves are toxic and contain oxalic acid, which can damage the kidneys when consumed in high amounts.

Pairs with: Strawberries, blueberries, sugar and other sweeteners, oats, lemons, red onions, and oranges.

Varieties: Can be predominantly red but also can be pink, green, or a combination of these colors.

Preparation: Use a knife to cut off the leaves and the ends of the stalks. Rinse under cold water to clean, and cut into ½-inch to 1-inch slices, similar to how you would prepare celery.

Favorite cooking methods: Baked into desserts, and cooked down into jams and chutneys.

Nutritional info: Rhubarb provides fiber, bone-building calcium, and vitamin K that assists in blood clotting. While plain rhubarb is very nutritious, most desserts that feature it are high in added sugar.

Selection: Rhubarb stalks should be firm, with healthy ends that do not look dried out. Floppy stalks are a sign that the rhubarb is old.

Storage: Store rhubarb stalks in a sealed bag or wrapped in plastic wrap in the refrigerator for up to 1 week. You can extend the short rhubarb season by buying in bulk and freezing for later. Cut the stalks into pieces, lay them on a plate, transfer to the freezer for a few hours until firm, then keep them in zip-top plastic freezer bags for several months.

Rhubarb and Candied Ginger Jam

Makes about 3 cups | Prep time: 25 minutes | Cook time: 20 minutes

This is a delicious spin on rhubarb jam! The spicy flavor of the ginger really wakes up your tastebuds for that sweet and refreshing bite.

4 cups sliced rhubarb, cut into ½-inch pieces

1½ cups granulated sugar

Zest and juice of 1 lemon

¼ cup finely chopped Homemade Candied Ginger (page 85)

1. In a large bowl, mix together the rhubarb, sugar, lemon zest, lemon juice, and ginger. Let sit until the rhubarb releases its juices, about 20 minutes.
2. Transfer the ingredients to a saucepan and bring to a boil, stirring frequently, over medium-high heat. Lower the heat to medium and simmer for 15 to 20 minutes, or until the jam thickens.
3. Transfer to glass jars, let the jam cool to room temperature, secure the lids tightly, and store in the refrigerator for up to 3 weeks. Serve on toast, biscuits, or crackers.

Rutabaga

Season: Fall and Winter

Flavor profile: Rutabagas, also known as swedes, taste like a cross between turnips and Yukon gold potatoes. Cooking transforms their slightly bitter flavor and brings out sweet and savory undertones. The texture of rutabaga is crispy like a carrot when raw, and creamy when cooked.

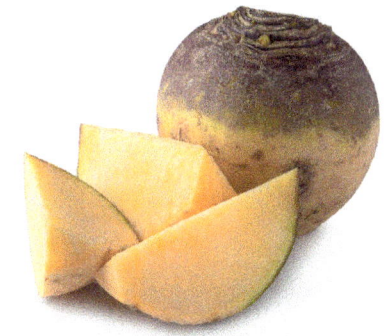

Pairs with: Apples, pears, onions, potatoes, carrots, garlic, mustard, walnuts, brown sugar, rosemary, and thyme.

Varieties: Several that all have a purple top and a golden yellow root.

Preparation: Trim the ends, scrub clean with a vegetable brush, peel if desired, and cut into pieces.

Favorite cooking methods: Grated or shaved, roasted, and mashed.

Nutritional info: Rutabagas are especially rich in anti-aging vitamin C, as well as potassium, magnesium, and calcium that work together to maintain healthy blood pressure.

Selection: Look for rutabagas that are firm and unblemished. While small cuts around the top are normal, rutabagas should not have large slashes on their skin.

Storage: Place rutabagas unwashed in a sealed plastic bag or container in the refrigerator. They typically last for 2 weeks or sometimes longer.

Shaved Rutabaga and Peanut Salad

Serves 4 | Prep time: 10 minutes

Rutabagas are a hearty, sweet root vegetable that tastes great raw in salads.

FOR THE SALAD

- 1 rutabaga, peeled and shaved into thin slices with a mandoline
- 2 scallions, thinly sliced
- ¼ cup chopped peanuts
- 2 tablespoons chopped fresh cilantro

FOR THE DRESSING

- 3 tablespoons extra-virgin olive oil
- 1 tablespoon rice vinegar
- Juice of 1 lime
- 2 teaspoons maple syrup

TO MAKE THE SALAD

1. In a large bowl, mix together the rutabaga, scallions, peanuts, and cilantro.

TO MAKE THE DRESSING

2. In a small bowl, whisk together the olive oil, vinegar, lime juice, and maple syrup until smooth.
3. Add the dressing to the salad and toss until evenly coated.

Spinach

Season: Spring and Fall

Flavor profile: Spinach has a grassy, earthy taste that's milder than peppery arugula or hearty kale. It is not as tough as some leafy greens, making it an ideal base for salads.

Pairs with: Olive oil, most vinegars, garlic, soy sauce, ginger, red pepper flakes, artichokes, and most fresh fruits.

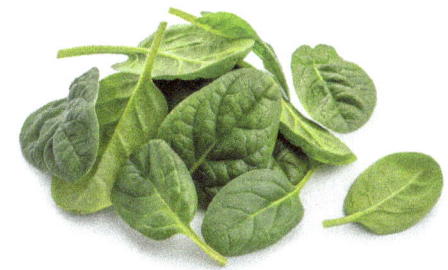

Varieties: Baby or mature flat-leaf and curly-leaf (known as savoy or semi-savoy).

Preparation: Rinse clean in a colander under cold water. Pat dry or use a salad spinner to get rid of excess water. Spinach can be chopped with a chef's knife or in a food processor.

Favorite cooking methods: Raw in salads, blended into smoothies, and sautéed.

Nutritional info: Not only is spinach a source of iron, calcium, folate, and vitamins A, C, and K, but it's also loaded with antioxidants such as quercetin and kaempferol.

Selection: Fresh spinach is bright green and crisp. Avoid leaves that are yellowed, wilted, or slimy.

Storage: Wrap unwashed spinach in paper towels to help absorb moisture and prolong its shelf life. Store in a plastic bag or in its original container for up to 5 days in the refrigerator.

Easy Wilted Spinach

Serves 4 | Prep time: 5 minutes | Cook time: 5 minutes

Spinach is great on its own, but gently wilting the leaves adds a whole new level. They become soft, juicy, and full of a unique savory flavor.

- 1 tablespoon extra-virgin olive oil
- 3 garlic cloves, minced
- 8 cups loosely packed spinach
- Salt
- Freshly ground black pepper
- 4 lemon wedges, for serving (optional)

1. In a large skillet over medium heat, warm the olive oil. Add the garlic and cook for 3 to 4 minutes, or until fragrant.
2. Add the spinach and cook for 3 to 5 minutes, or until wilted. Season with salt and pepper. Sprinkle with freshly squeezed lemon juice just before serving if desired.

Spinach and White Bean Stir-Fry

Serves 4 | Prep time: 5 minutes | Cook time: 15 minutes

Since sautéed spinach cooks down quickly, you can pack a ton of this nutritious green into stir-fries. With a touch of coconut, spicy red pepper flakes, creamy white beans, and chewy farro, eating your greens has never been this delicious. Bookmark this easy vegetarian main dish for when you have a hankering for a fast meal that's still healthy and tasty.

1 tablespoon extra-virgin olive oil

3 garlic cloves, minced

8 cups loosely packed spinach

¼ cup plain full-fat coconut milk

1 tablespoon soy sauce

⅛ to ¼ teaspoon red pepper flakes

1 (15-ounce) can white beans, drained and rinsed

2 cups cooked farro, for serving

1. In a large skillet over medium heat, warm the olive oil. Add the garlic and cook for 3 to 4 minutes, or until fragrant.
2. Add the spinach, coconut milk, soy sauce, and red pepper flakes, stir to combine, and cook for 3 to 5 minutes, or until the spinach is wilted.
3. Add the white beans to the skillet and cook for 3 to 4 minutes, or until warmed through.
4. Divide the farro among four shallow bowls. Top with the spinach mixture, spoon any remaining sauce over the top, and serve.

Notes: Prep the farro in advance to have on hand for when you make this dish. You can find quick-cooking farro at Trader Joe's and some other stores. Substitute tamari for the soy sauce to make this dish gluten-free.

Sprouts and Microgreens

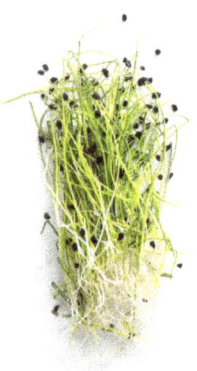 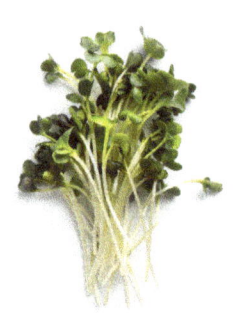

Season: Any (can grow indoors)

Flavor profile: Microgreens can be sweet and mild, with a slightly nutty flavor.

Pairs with: Sprouted microgreens are perfect for salads, sandwiches, and even raw.

Varieties: You can sprout most greens and veggies.

Preparation: Simply grow them in your garden or indoors, and enjoy raw. No real preparation is required.

Favorite cooking methods: Best eaten raw.

Nutritional info: Sprouts are loaded with vitamins and minerals, such as vitamins A and C, calcium, iron, and protein.

Selection: Select sprouts that are bright in color and look vibrant.

Storage: Keep sprouts stored in your refrigerator.

Citrusy Microgreens

Serves 4 | Prep time: 5 minutes

As their name suggests, microgreens are tiny greens that grow from the seeds of vegetables and herbs. Despite their small size, they're rich in nutrients and can be a versatile ingredient. Toss microgreens in freshly squeezed orange and lemon juices for a healthy side salad or garnish. You can even serve this recipe on top of toast with hummus or ricotta for a quick breakfast or lunch.

2 tablespoons extra-virgin olive oil

1 tablespoon freshly squeezed lemon juice, plus more as needed

1 tablespoon freshly squeezed orange juice, plus more as needed

2 cups microgreens

½ cup salted sunflower seeds

Salt

1. In a bowl, whisk together the olive oil, lemon juice, and orange juice.
2. Add the microgreens and sunflower seeds. Toss until evenly coated. Season with salt. Taste and add more citrus juices as needed.

Notes: The microgreens taste best when enjoyed right away, since they can get soggy after sitting in the dressing. Add some orange or lemon zest in addition to the juice for more flavor.

Sweet Potatoes

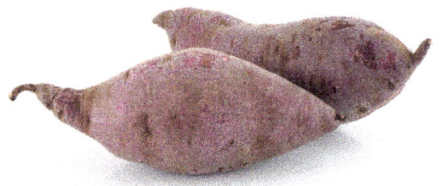

Season: Fall and Winter

Flavor profile: As their name suggests, sweet potatoes have a deliciously sweet taste that's reminiscent of some winter squashes. When cooked, they have creamy flesh and a buttery mouthfeel.

Pairs with: Rosemary, sage, cinnamon, ginger, coconut, chili powder, paprika, apples, onions, walnuts, and pecans.

Varieties: Orange, yellow, red, white, or purple skin with orange, yellow, or white flesh.

Preparation: Scrub clean with a vegetable brush, and use a swivel peeler to remove the skin if desired. Roast whole or cut into pieces.

Favorite cooking methods: Roasted, mashed, stuffed, and made into noodles.

Nutritional info: Sweet potatoes are known for being an extremely good source of beta-carotene, the pigment that's responsible for their orange flesh and gets converted into vitamin A in the body. Consuming enough vitamin A is vital to maintaining good eyesight.

Selection: Choose firm sweet potatoes with smooth skin that's not cracked. Small or medium sweet potatoes tend to be sweeter than larger ones.

Storage: Keep sweet potatoes in a cool, dry, and dark place. Use within 2 weeks.

Sweet Potato and Chickpea Curry

Serves 4 | Prep time: 5 minutes | Cook time: 25 minutes

Curry is the best kind of vegetarian meal: full of flavor and so easy to prepare. In this version, tender sweet potatoes are simmered in a luscious coconut-based sauce. Enjoy this comforting meal for dinner on a cold night and have the leftovers for lunch the next day . . . or not. I have a feeling you'll be hurrying back for seconds with this one.

2 tablespoons coconut oil
1 yellow onion, diced
3 garlic cloves, minced
1 sweet potato, diced
2 teaspoons curry powder
1 teaspoon ground cumin
½ teaspoon ground ginger
2 cups vegetable broth
1 (13.5-ounce) can full-fat coconut milk
1 (15-ounce) can chickpeas, drained and rinsed

1. In a large skillet over medium heat, warm the coconut oil. Add the onion and garlic and cook for 3 to 4 minutes, or until fragrant.

2. Add the sweet potato, curry powder, cumin, ginger, and broth and stir to combine. Reduce the heat to medium-low, cover, and simmer for about 10 minutes, or until the potatoes are almost tender.

3. Add the coconut milk and chickpeas, raise the heat to medium, and cook, uncovered, stirring occasionally, for another 8 to 10 minutes, or until the curry begins to thicken. Serve warm.

Notes: Enjoy this curry on its own or with naan bread and/or rice. Use curry paste in lieu of curry powder for an even spicier dish.

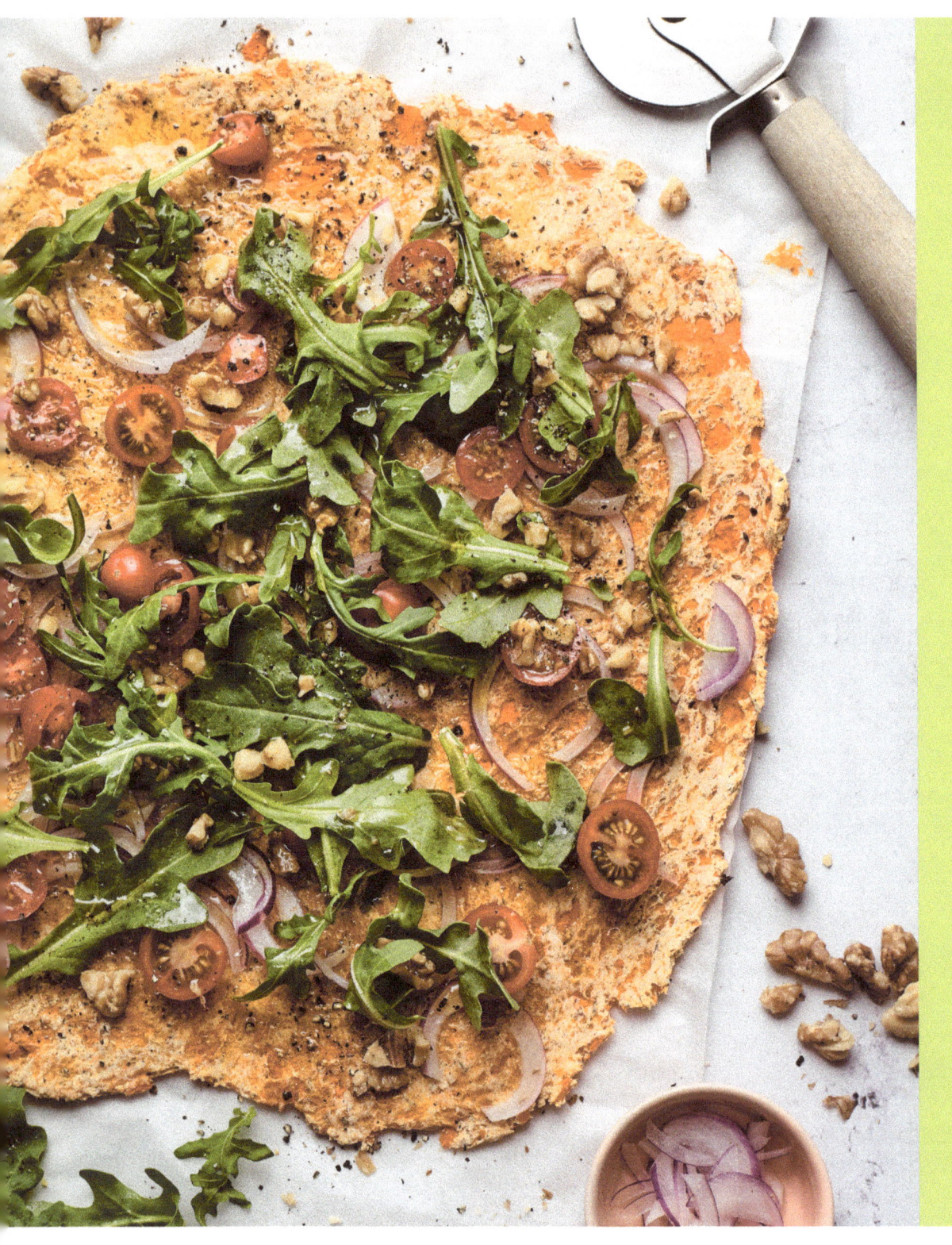

Sweet Potato Pizza Crust

Serves 4 | Prep time: 20 minutes | Cook time: 20 minutes

Using only five ingredients, this pizza crust takes only 20 minutes to make and the same amount of time to bake. Best of all, it's not overly sweet and won't fall apart in the oven. Once you've baked the crust, cover it with your favorite pizza toppings for a delicious dinner.

2 cups water

2 sweet potatoes, peeled and chopped

1 cup all-purpose flour or gluten-free flour

¼ cup cornstarch

2 tablespoons flaxseed meal

½ teaspoon salt

1. Preheat the oven to 425°F. Line a baking sheet with parchment paper.

2. In a medium saucepan, bring the water to a boil over high heat. Add the sweet potatoes to the boiling water and cook for 15 minutes, or until the potatoes are soft.

3. Drain and let cool, then transfer to a bowl and mash.

4. Measure out 2 cups of the mashed sweet potato and transfer it to a large bowl (save any extra for another use). Add the flour, cornstarch, flaxseed meal, and salt. Mix well.

5. Transfer the dough to the center of the prepared baking sheet. Using another piece of parchment paper, press down on the dough gently with your hands to flatten it into an even circle. Peel off the top sheet of parchment paper and bake for 20 minutes.

Sweet Potato Gnocchi

Serves 2 | Prep time: 20 minutes | Cook time: 5 minutes

Making your own gnocchi is surprisingly easy but extremely satisfying. Using sweet potato instead of potato adds a gentle sweetness that is a great match for pretty much any sauce, whether it's marinara, pesto, or a vegan cream.

2 large sweet potatoes, peeled

1 cup whole-wheat flour or gluten-free flour, plus more for kneading

½ cup brown rice flour

3 garlic cloves, finely minced

Pinch Himalayan salt

Pinch pepper

1. Boil a large pot of water. Pierce the sweet potatoes with a fork in several places, then boil them until tender. Remove them from the water and let them cool.
2. Once the sweet potatoes are cool, place the boiled sweet potatoes, whole-wheat flour, rice flour, garlic, salt, and pepper in a food processor. Pulse until well combined.
3. Transfer the mixture to a well-floured flat surface and knead into a dough ball.
4. Divide the dough into roughly 8 equal parts. Roll each part into a log about ½-inch thick, then cut the log into 1-inch pieces.
5. Using your finger, slightly press each piece at the center to give it a pillowy shape.
6. Cook the prepared gnocchi in boiling water for 5 minutes, or until they start to float on the surface.

Notes: Serve with olive oil, sautéed mushrooms, and steamed kale, or your preferred sauce.

Tomatillos

Season: Summer and Fall

Flavor profile: Tomatillos are commonly used in Mexican and South American cooking. The small green fruits have a lemon, citrus, sweet, tart flavor.

Pairs with: Salsa, chipotle, and soups.

Varieties: Amarylla, Gigante, Green Husk, Mexican, Pineapple, Purple de Milpa, and Yellow.

Preparation: Peel the husks and give the tomatillos a rinse in a colander to remove any sticky residue.

Favorite cooking methods: Chopped raw for salsa, boiled, and slow-cooked.

Nutritional info: Tomatillos are low in calories and a good source of iron, magnesium, phosphorus, copper, vitamin C, and vitamin K.

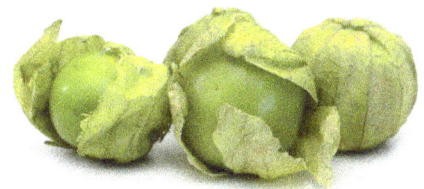

Selection: For a sweeter flavor, look for overripe fruit that will be pale yellow or light green. Pick a tomatillo that has a bright green husk.

Storage: Store in your refrigerator or freezer or use right away. They can last on your counter for about 2 days.

Posole Verde

Serves 4 | Prep time: 10 minutes | Cook time: 40 minutes

Pinto beans, hominy, tomatillos, and jalapeño join forces in this tasty and vibrant main dish that works just as well for a hearty lunch as it does for dinner. Brimming with zesty flavor, it's a treat for your tastebuds.

1 tablespoon extra-virgin olive oil

1 large onion, diced

1 large jalapeño, diced

4 large garlic cloves, minced

1 teaspoon cumin

1 teaspoon oregano

Salt

Freshly ground black pepper

2 (15-ounce) cans pinto beans, drained and rinsed

1 (15-ounce) can hominy, drained and rinsed

6 medium tomatillos, husked, well rinsed, and chopped

4 cups vegetable broth

Juice of 2 limes

1. In a large pot, warm the oil over medium heat. Add the onion and sauté for 5 minutes.
2. Add the jalapeño, garlic, cumin, oregano, salt, and pepper, then cook for another minute, or until fragrant.
3. Add the pinto beans, hominy, tomatillos, and broth. Bring to a boil, cover, reduce the heat to low, and simmer for 30 minutes.
4. Add the lime juice and season to taste.

Tomatoes

Season: Summer

Flavor profile: Even though they are technically considered fruits, tomatoes are often grouped with vegetables for culinary purposes. They have juicy flesh and a sweet, acidic taste that's slightly different for each variety.

Pairs with: Garlic, onions, olive oil, basil, thyme, chives, parsley, cilantro, red pepper flakes, and stone fruits.

Varieties: Beefsteak, heirloom, San Marzano, cherry or grape, and several other varieties that can be red, green, or yellow-orange.

Preparation: Remove the stems, wash, and pat dry. Use a serrated knife to cut tomatoes.

Favorite cooking methods: Raw, grilled, and blended into sauces or soups.

Nutritional info: Tomatoes provide a variety of nutrients and health-promoting compounds, including the red pigment lycopene. This antioxidant may help lower blood pressure and prevent the buildup of plaque in arteries.

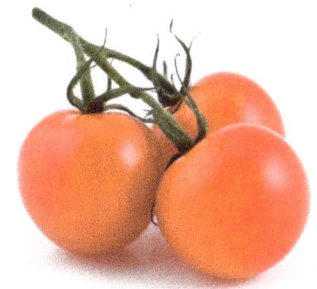

Selection: Look for tomatoes that are plump, smooth, and free of cracks or dark spots. To truly test their freshness, pick up tomatoes and smell them to ensure that they have a sweet, earthy fragrance.

Storage: Place ripe or almost ripe tomatoes on a plate and store at room temperature away from direct sunlight for a few days. Overripe tomatoes can be refrigerated to prevent rotting but should be used within 2 days.

Homemade Tomato Sauce

Makes about 3 cups | Prep time: 5 minutes | Cook time: 20 minutes

Making tomato sauce from scratch may sound intimidating, but as soon as you see how easy it is, you'll wonder why you haven't tried it sooner. The key to a truly delicious sauce is using San Marzano tomatoes, which are known for their sweetness and low acidity. Once you have the proper ingredients, the stovetop does the rest of the work. If you go through a lot of tomato sauce in your house, I recommend making this recipe in bulk and freezing for later.

2 tablespoons extra-virgin olive oil

4 garlic cloves, minced

1 (28-ounce) can whole peeled San Marzano tomatoes

½ teaspoon salt, plus more as needed

Freshly ground black pepper

1. In a saucepan over medium-low heat, warm the olive oil. Add the garlic and cook, stirring frequently to avoid burning, for 2 to 3 minutes, or until the garlic is fragrant.
2. Add the tomatoes along with their juices and the salt. Simmer, using a wooden spoon to crush the tomatoes as they cook, for 15 to 20 minutes, or until the sauce has reached your desired thickness. Season with salt and pepper to taste.
3. Use immediately or transfer to glass jars, let cool, and store in the refrigerator for up to 1 week.

Notes: To freeze this sauce, let it cool to room temperature before transferring to freezer-safe containers. It will last for at least 3 months in the freezer. Thaw in the refrigerator before using. To make this more like a marinara sauce, add up to 1 teaspoon each of dried basil and oregano and a pinch of red pepper flakes for some spice.

Garden Tomato Soup

Serves 4 to 6 | Prep time: 10 minutes | Cook time: 25 minutes

If there was ever a recipe for your late summer garden overflowing with tomatoes, it's this one. Instead of the canned tomatoes that are typically used in classic tomato soup, I like to throw in the freshest, juiciest tomatoes I can find in my backyard or at the farmers' market. Any variety works.

- 2 tablespoons extra-virgin olive oil
- 1 sweet onion, diced
- 3 garlic cloves, minced
- 4 cups chopped fresh tomatoes with their juices
- 1 teaspoon tomato paste
- 2 cups vegetable broth
- ½ teaspoon salt, plus more as needed
- ¼ teaspoon freshly ground black pepper, plus more as needed
- 1 or 2 tablespoons chiffonaded fresh basil, for serving

1. In a large pot over medium heat, warm the olive oil. Add the onion and garlic and cook for 3 to 4 minutes, or until fragrant.
2. Add the chopped tomatoes and tomato paste and cook for another 5 to 7 minutes.
3. Add the broth, salt, and pepper and simmer for about 15 minutes.
4. Using an immersion blender, puree the soup in the pot. Taste and adjust the seasonings as desired.
5. Serve warm with a sprinkle of fresh basil.

Notes: To blend the soup safely in a regular blender, fill it halfway and puree the soup in batches. Leave a corner of the lid cracked, or remove the top of the blender and cover it with a folded dish towel to let steam escape as you blend. Be careful not to get burned by the steam.

Turnips

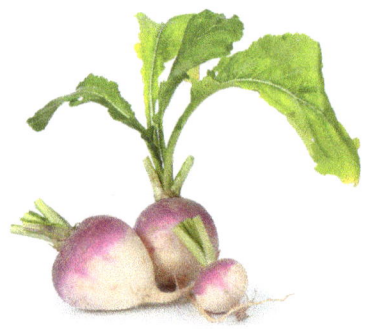

Season: Fall and Winter

Flavor profile: Turnips are a crunchy root vegetable with a pungent taste that's mildly bitter and spicy. Cooking helps mellow their flavor, and younger turnips are generally sweeter than more mature ones. Turnip greens are also edible and taste similar to the roots.

Pairs with: Mustard, sage, rosemary, chives, thyme, garlic, apples, carrots, beets, and potatoes.

Varieties: Purple-top, baby, white, and scarlet.

Preparation: Scrub clean with a vegetable brush, peel if desired, and dice.

Favorite cooking methods: Grated or shaved, roasted, mashed, and made into noodles.

Nutritional info: Turnips are part of the cruciferous vegetable family and may provide health benefits similar to those of kale, Brussels sprouts, and bok choy. They are rich in both vitamin C and glucosinolates, compounds that may prevent cancer cell growth.

Selection: Turnips should be firm and heavy. Their skin should be smooth and free of cracks.

Storage: Keep whole, unwashed turnips in a plastic bag or airtight container in the refrigerator for 2 weeks or longer.

Maple-Mustard Roasted Turnips

Serves 4 | Prep time: 5 minutes | Cook time: 30 minutes

The sweetness of the maple syrup, the zest of the mustard, and the roasted flavor of the turnips will make these the highlight of any meal! The combination of sweet and savory at its finest.

2 tablespoons maple syrup

1 tablespoon Dijon mustard

1 tablespoon extra-virgin olive oil

2 large turnips, peeled and diced

Salt

Chopped fresh parsley or thyme, for serving (optional)

1. Preheat the oven to 400°F. Line a baking sheet with parchment paper.

2. In a medium bowl, stir together the maple syrup, mustard, and olive oil. Add the diced turnips and toss until evenly coated. Spread the turnips in a single layer on the baking sheet, and season with salt.

3. Roast, flipping halfway through, for 30 to 35 minutes, or until tender. Garnish with fresh parsley or thyme if desired.

Pureed Turnip and Garlic Dip

Makes about 3 cups | Prep time: 10 minutes | Cook time: 30 minutes

Roasting root vegetables brings out their natural sweetness, and roasted turnips are no exception. Turnips also take on a tender, buttery texture when cooked, making them an ideal base for creamy dips. This healthy snack pairs mellowed turnips with roasted garlic. It's zesty, nutritious, and a great companion to seed crackers or tortilla chips.

3 cups diced turnips

3 tablespoons extra-virgin olive oil, divided

Salt

Freshly ground black pepper

3 or 4 cloves from a Roasted Garlic Bulb (page 82)

Juice of ½ lemon

Toasted sesame seeds, for serving

1. Preheat the oven to 400°F. Line a baking sheet with parchment paper.
2. Place the turnips on the prepared baking sheet, toss with 1 tablespoon of olive oil, and season with salt and pepper. Bake for about 30 minutes, or until tender.
3. In a food processor or high-powered blender, combine the roasted turnips, garlic, lemon juice, and remaining 2 tablespoons of olive oil, and season with salt and pepper. Pulse until smooth. Taste and adjust the seasonings as needed.
4. Transfer to a serving bowl and top with toasted sesame seeds.

Notes: While cloves from a whole roasted garlic bulb add more creamy texture and flavor, you can also roast the garlic cloves with the turnips if you're short on time. Store the dip for up to 1 week in an airtight container in the refrigerator.

Winter Squash

Season: Fall and Winter

Flavor profile: From the sweet flavor of butternut to the earthy, nutty palate of acorn, winter squashes vary in taste. In general, the flesh of cooked squash is rich and creamy with subtly sweet undertones.

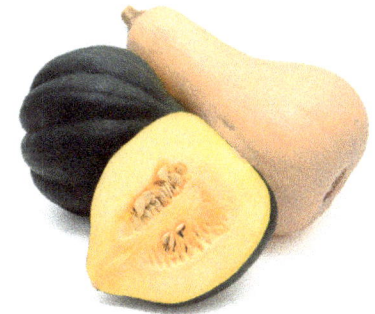

Pairs with: Rosemary, sage, thyme, cinnamon, cloves, allspice, nutmeg, ginger, apples, pears, and cranberries.

Varieties: Acorn, butternut, delicata, hubbard, kabocha, pumpkin, red kuri, and spaghetti squash.

Preparation: Use a chef's knife to remove the top and stem. Cut in half lengthwise from top to bottom, scoop out the seeds with a spoon, and remove the skin with a swivel peeler or knife. Cut into desired shapes. If the squash is difficult to cut, make several slits with a knife on the part of the skin where you want to cut it in half. Microwave on high for 3 to 4 minutes to soften the skin.

Favorite cooking methods: Roasted, stuffed, and pureed.

Nutritional info: The nutrition of each type of winter squash varies, but they are all rich in fiber and micronutrients. Most squash provide generous amounts of antioxidant carotenoids that are responsible for their bright-colored flesh.

Selection: Pick up the squash to ensure that it feels heavy and has a smooth surface without cracks or bruises. Squash stems should be dry and firm.

Storage: Winter squash will keep for at least a few weeks when stored in a cool, dry place.

Acorn Squash with Cranberry and Wild Rice Stuffing

Serves 4 | Prep time: 15 minutes | Cook time: 45 minutes

I had never cooked with wild rice until I moved to Minnesota, where it is the official state grain. Now, I can't get enough of this nutty, protein-rich grain that pairs especially well with acorn squash. With bright red cranberries and green sage, this recipe for stuffed squash can serve as a festive vegetarian main dish for Thanksgiving or Christmas.

FOR THE SQUASH

- 2 acorn squash, halved lengthwise and seeded
- 1 teaspoon extra-virgin olive oil
- Salt
- Freshly ground black pepper

FOR THE STUFFING

- 1 cup wild rice
- 3 cups vegetable broth
- 1 tablespoon extra-virgin olive oil
- 1 yellow onion, diced
- 16 ounces cremini mushrooms, thinly sliced
- 1 cup fresh cranberries
- 2 tablespoons chopped fresh sage

TO MAKE THE SQUASH

1. Preheat the oven to 400°F. Line a baking sheet with parchment paper.
2. Brush the cut sides of the squash with olive oil and season with salt and pepper. Bake for 30 to 35 minutes, or until tender.

TO MAKE THE STUFFING

3. While the squash is roasting, in a saucepan over high heat, combine the wild rice and broth and bring to a boil. Reduce the heat to medium-low, cover with a loose-fitting lid, and simmer for 25 to 35 minutes, or until tender.
4. In a large skillet over medium heat, warm the olive oil. Add the onion and mushrooms and cook for 6 to 8 minutes, or until softened.
5. Add the cranberries and sage and cook for another 5 minutes, or until the cranberries begin to pop. Remove from the heat, add the cooked wild rice, and stir to combine.
6. Stuff each squash half with a generous spoonful of the wild rice and cranberry mixture and serve.

Notes: Some varieties of wild rice take longer to cook, so refer to the package instructions before making it. Cook the rice in advance to cut down on prep time. If you can't find fresh cranberries, substitute ½ cup of dried cranberries.

Spaghetti Squash with Kale and Chickpeas

Serves 2 | Prep time: 10 minutes | Cook time: 50 minutes

Spaghetti squash is a satisfying alternative to pasta noodles. The strands look exactly like spaghetti noodles and have a mild nutty flavor that goes well with any kind of sauce or topping. This recipe calls for a light olive oil sauce with lemon, chickpeas, kale, sun-dried tomatoes, and pine nuts.

1 spaghetti squash

Sea salt

Freshly ground black pepper

2 tablespoons extra-virgin olive oil

2 shallots, thinly sliced

2 garlic cloves

½ tablespoon minced fresh rosemary

Pinch chili flakes

½ cup cooked chickpeas, drained and rinsed

2 packed cups chopped kale leaves

1 tablespoon lemon juice

¼ cup chopped sun-dried tomatoes

¼ cup toasted pine nuts

1. Preheat the oven to 350°F.
2. Cut the squash in half lengthwise and scoop out the seeds. Sprinkle the inside with salt and pepper. Roast for 40 minutes, or until lightly browned on the outside.
3. Remove the squash from oven and let cool, then use a fork to scrape the strands from the inside.
4. In a large skillet over medium heat, warm the olive oil. Add the shallots, whole garlic cloves, rosemary, chili flakes, and salt and pepper, and cook until the shallots start to soften.
5. Add the chickpeas and cook for 2 to 3 minutes, until lightly golden brown.
6. Add the kale and lemon juice, stir, and cook until the kale is partially wilted.
7. Add the squash strands, sun-dried tomatoes, and more salt and pepper, to taste. Toss to incorporate.
8. Remove from the heat and top with the toasted pine nuts.

Pumpkin Pasta Carbonara

Serves 2 | Prep time: 15 minutes | Cook time: 40 minutes

The Italian classic carbonara recipe meets pumpkin for a silky pasta dish. The sage adds an amazing aroma and pine flavor, while the coconut yogurt is both cooling and creamy, blending harmoniously with the pumpkin. This will likely become a fall staple in your household.

2 tablespoons extra-virgin olive oil

½ cup fresh sage leaves

1 white onion, diced

2 garlic cloves, thinly sliced

1 small pumpkin, peeled and cut into small cubes

2 cups unsweetened plant milk

¼ teaspoon red chili flakes

½ teaspoon cracked black pepper

½ teaspoon Himalayan sea salt

1 box rigatoni pasta

¼ cup natural coconut yogurt

1 tablespoon nutritional yeast

1. In a deep saucepan over medium-high heat, warm the olive oil. Add the sage and sauté for 6 minutes. Remove the sage and set aside.
2. Keeping the saucepan over the heat, add the onion and garlic and sauté for 4 minutes, or until soft and golden.
3. Add the pumpkin and plant milk to the pan and simmer uncovered for 30 minutes, or until the pumpkin is soft. Add the chili flakes, pepper, and salt.
4. Cook the pasta according to the package instructions. Drain and set aside in a saucepan.
5. Transfer the pumpkin mixture to a blender or use an immersion blender to puree until smooth. Add the yogurt and nutritional yeast and blend to combine well.
6. Stir the sauce through the pasta over medium-low heat until well combined and heated through. Top with the sage.

Zucchini and Summer Squash

Season: Summer

Flavor profile: With a fairly bland flavor and spongy flesh, zucchini and yellow squash absorb seasonings very well. Their sweet and floral undertones are very subtle.

Pairs with: Tomatoes, eggplant, garlic, onions, basil, oregano, soy sauce, red pepper flakes, ginger, chocolate, bananas, and oats.

Varieties: Green zucchini, yellow crookneck, pattypan, and several others.

Preparation: Trim the stems and ends. Use a swivel peeler to remove the skin if desired. Cut into the desired size or run through a spiralizer.

Favorite cooking methods: Sautéed, roasted, made into noodles, and shredded into baked goods.

Nutritional info: Summer squashes are low in calories but high in water and fiber. Adding them to your diet can help promote healthy digestion.

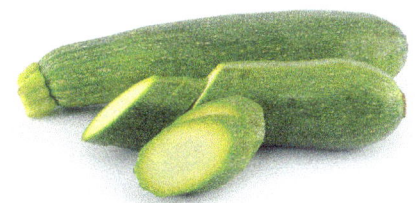

Selection: Choose zucchini and summer squash that are firm, bright in color, and free of scratches. The skin should not be shriveled or spotted.

Storage: Place whole, unwashed zucchini in a perforated plastic bag in the produce drawer of the refrigerator. They can be stored for up to 2 weeks.

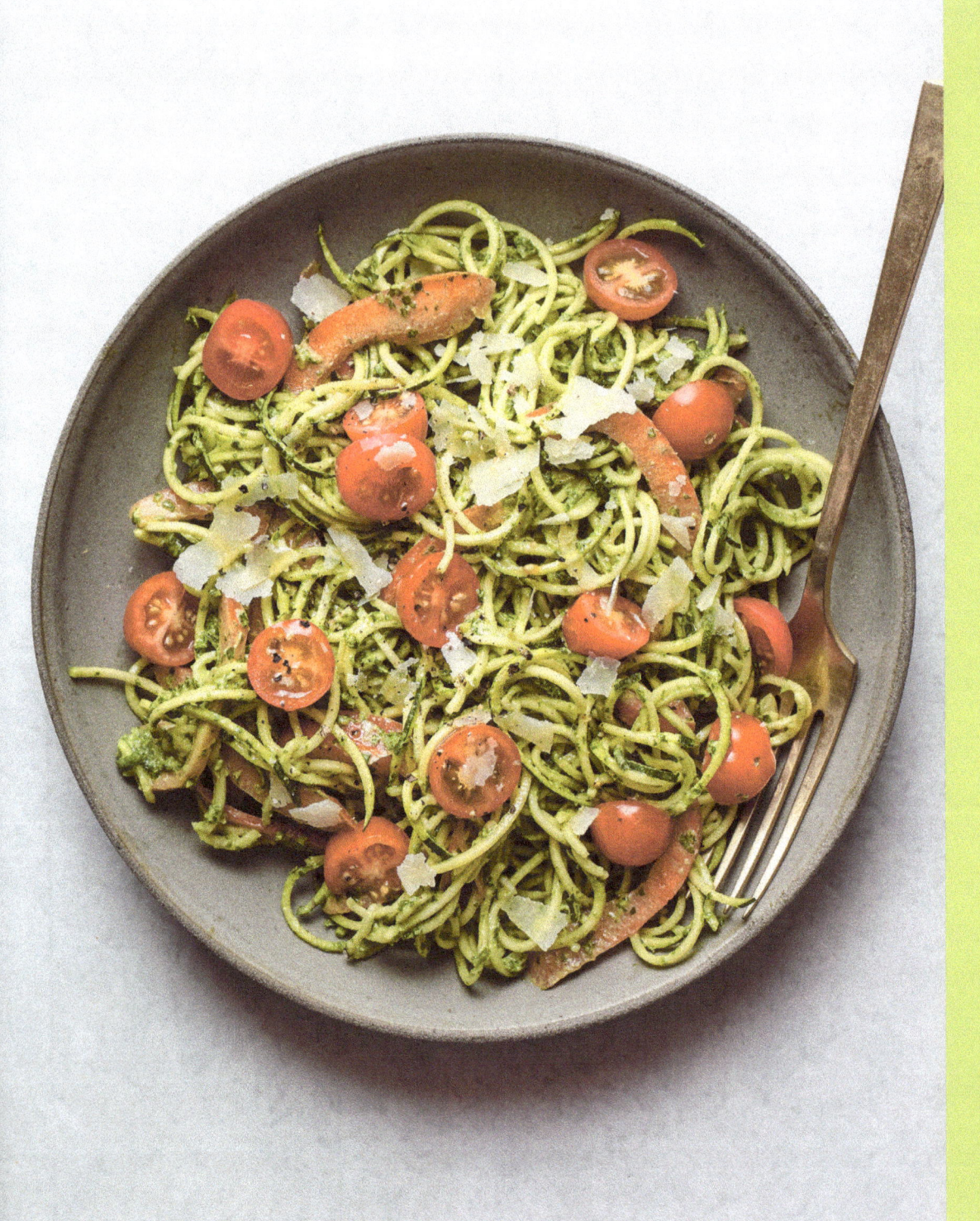

Zucchini Pesto Pasta

Serves 2 Prep time: 10 minutes

Creating zoodles using a spiralizer is my go-to pasta replacement. This dish pairs the zoodles with a light homemade tahini pesto and bell peppers for added sweetness. It's a great meal for a hot summer day, giving you the pasta experience without the heaviness.

4 zucchini

3 cups fresh basil

2 garlic cloves

3 tablespoons tahini

½ teaspoon salt

1 yellow bell pepper, thinly sliced

Halved cherry tomatoes, for serving

Freshly shaved vegan Parmesan cheese, for serving

1. Use a spiralizer to create zoodles from the zucchini.
2. Combine the basil, garlic, tahini, and salt in a food processor and blend.
3. In a bowl, mix together the zoodles and bell pepper with the pesto.
4. Serve with halved cherry tomatoes and freshly shaved cheese.

Zucchini Boats

Serves 4 | Prep time: 15 minutes | Cook time: 45 minutes

Hearty yet light and full of veggies, these zucchini boats are both fun and filling. The savory marinara sauce and vegan sausage make this dish substantial enough to be served as an entrée, but the boats also work well as an accompanying dish.

4 medium zucchini

½ teaspoon sea salt

½ teaspoon garlic powder

Pinch red pepper flakes, plus ¼ teaspoon, and more as needed

2 tablespoons avocado oil

½ cup diced white onion

4 garlic cloves, minced

1¼ cups vegan sausage

1 cup marinara sauce

3 tablespoons grated vegan Parmesan cheese, plus more as needed

1. Preheat the oven to 400°F.
2. Cut the zucchini in half lengthwise and use a spoon to scoop out the seeds and some of the flesh. Sprinkle the boats with the salt, garlic powder, and a pinch of red pepper flakes.
3. Heat a large skillet on medium-high. Place the zucchini in the skillet cut-side down and cook for 3 minutes, or until the edges appear browned. After all the zucchini are seared, transfer to a baking dish cut-side up.
4. In the same skillet over medium heat, heat the avocado oil. Add the onion, garlic, and remaining ¼ teaspoon of red pepper flakes and sauté for 4 minutes, or until browned and translucent.
5. Add the vegan sausage and break up into small chunks. Cook, stirring frequently, for 10 minutes, or until the sausage has begun to brown. Remove from the heat and set aside.
6. Spoon the marinara sauce into the scooped-out part of the zucchini so that it's covered, and top with the vegan sausage mixture.
7. Top with the vegan cheese and bake uncovered for 25 minutes, or until the zucchini is tender. Serve immediately.

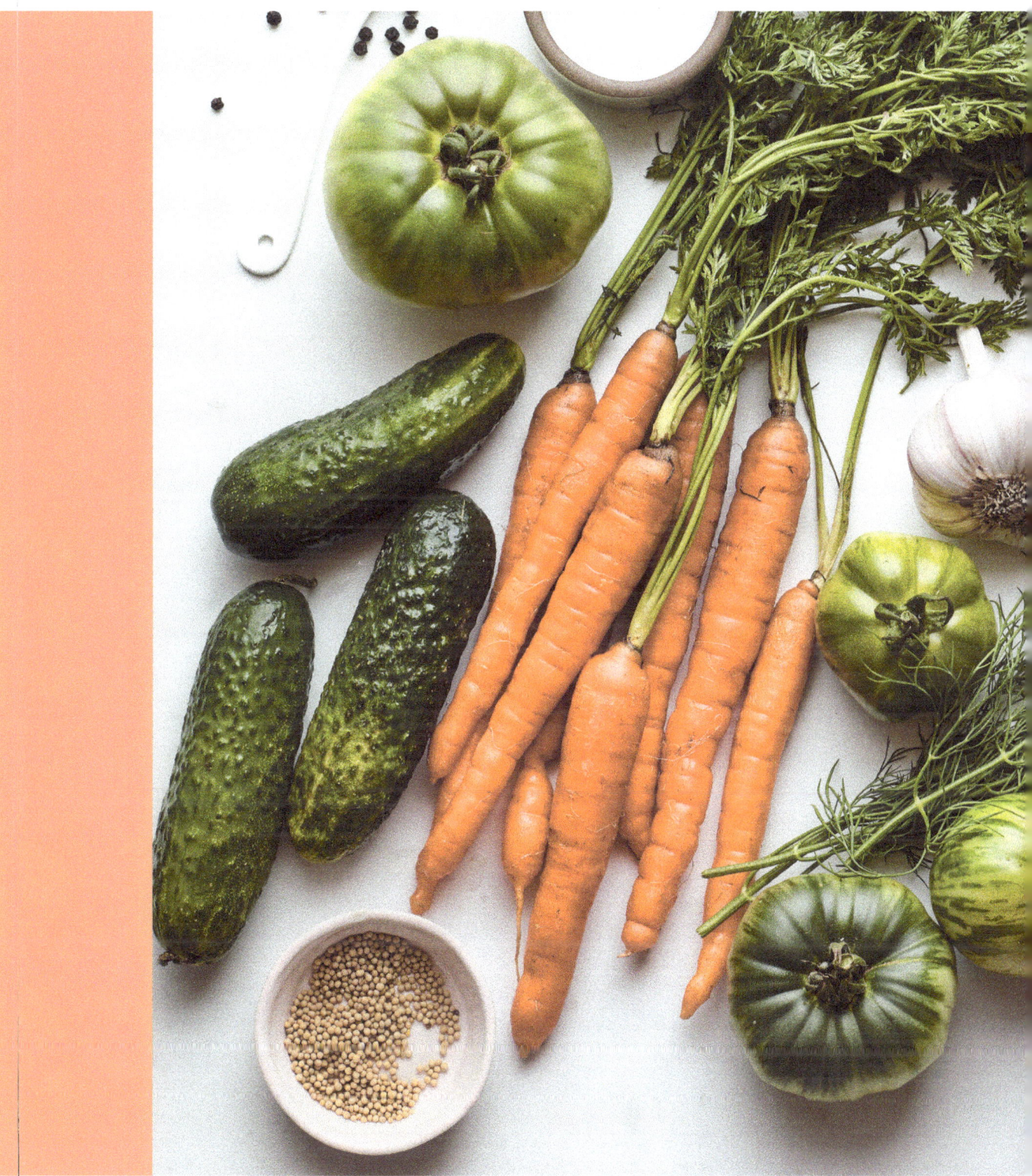

Carrots, p. 46

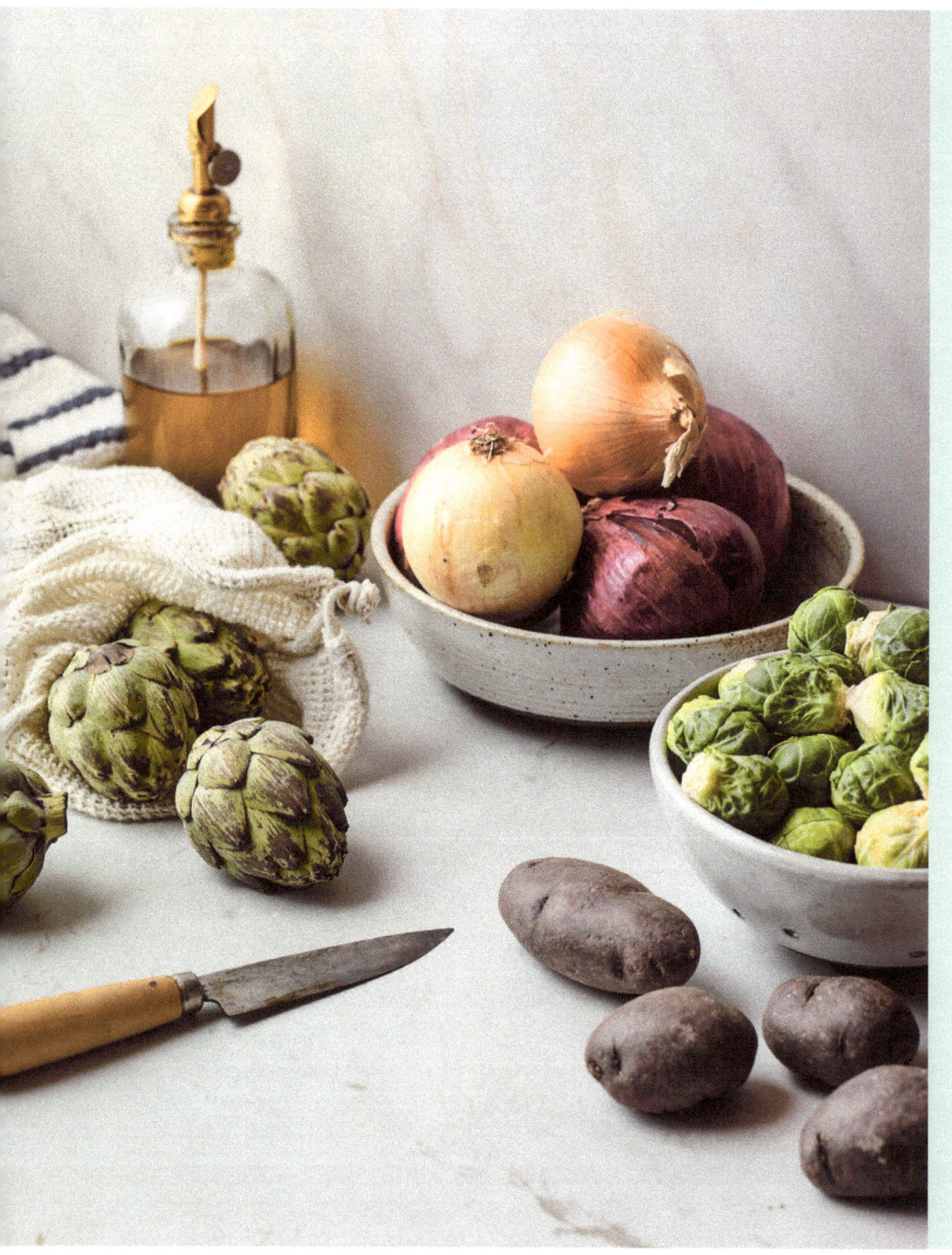

MEASUREMENT CONVERSIONS

	US STANDARD	US STANDARD (OUNCES)	METRIC (APPROXIMATE)
VOLUME EQUIVALENTS (LIQUID)	2 tablespoons	1 fl. oz.	30 mL
	¼ cup	2 fl. oz.	60 mL
	½ cup	4 fl. oz.	120 mL
	1 cup	8 fl. oz.	240 mL
	1½ cups	12 fl. oz.	355 mL
	2 cups or 1 pint	16 fl. oz.	475 mL
	4 cups or 1 quart	32 fl. oz.	1 L
	1 gallon	128 fl. oz.	4 L
VOLUME EQUIVALENTS (DRY)	⅛ teaspoon	—	0.5 mL
	¼ teaspoon	—	1 mL
	½ teaspoon	—	2 mL
	¾ teaspoon	—	4 mL
	1 teaspoon	—	5 mL
	1 tablespoon	—	15 mL
	¼ cup	—	59 mL
	⅓ cup	—	79 mL
	½ cup	—	118 mL
	⅔ cup	—	156 mL
	¾ cup	—	177 mL
	1 cup	—	235 mL
	2 cups or 1 pint	—	475 mL
	3 cups	—	700 mL
	4 cups or 1 quart	—	1 L
	½ gallon	—	2 L
	1 gallon	—	4 L
WEIGHT EQUIVALENTS	½ ounce	—	15 g
	1 ounce	—	30 g
	2 ounces	—	60 g
	4 ounces	—	115 g
	8 ounces	—	225 g
	12 ounces	—	340 g
	16 ounces or 1 pound	—	455 g

	FAHRENHEIT (F)	CELSIUS (C) (APPROXIMATE)
OVEN TEMPERATURES	250°F	120°C
	300°F	150°C
	325°F	180°C
	375°F	190°C
	400°F	200°C
	425°F	220°C
	450°F	230°C

INDEX

A

Acorn Squash with Cranberry and Wild Rice Stuffing, 164
Almond Butter and Pomegranate Arils, Celery with, 55
Apples
    Braised Cabbage, Apples, and White Beans, 44
    Parsnip and Apple Soup, 125
Artichokes
    about, 10
    Roasted Baby Artichokes, 13
    Simple Steamed Artichokes, 11
Arugula
    about, 14
    Arugula Salsa Verde, 15
    Sautéed Arugula with Roasted Red Peppers, 16
Asparagus
    about, 17
    Asparagus Soup with Peas, 19
    Linguine with Asparagus, 20
    Shaved Asparagus and Pine Nut Salad, 18
Avocados
    about, 21
    Avocado Toast with Quick Pickled Red Onions, 23
    Pineapple Avocado Salad, 22

B

Bacon, Eggplant, 70
Balsamic Roasted Mushrooms, 112
Beans. *See also* Fava beans; Green beans
    Braised Cabbage, Apples, and White Beans, 44
    Escarole and White Bean Soup, 62
    Kohlrabi Noodles with Red Sauce and Kidney Beans, 103
    Posole Verde, 156
    Spinach and White Bean Stir-Fry, 147
Beets
    about, 24
    Beet Fries with Garlic Tahini, 27
    Coconut Curry Golden Beet Soup, 25
Bell peppers
    about, 129
    Fresh Bell Pepper and Herb Salad, 131
    Roasted Red Peppers, 130
    Sautéed Arugula with Roasted Red Peppers, 16
    Stuffed Pepper Soup, 132
Bok choy
    about, 28
    Roasted Baby Bok Choy with Spicy Maple Miso, 30
    Sautéed Bok Choy, 29
Braising, 5
Broccoli
    about, 31
    Cilantro-Lime Riced Broccoli, 32
    Steamed Broccoli with Peanut Sauce, 33
    Teriyaki Tofu and Roasted Broccoli, 34
Broccoli rabe
    about, 37
    Classic Sautéed Broccoli Rabe, 38
Broccolini
    about, 35
    Broccolini Pasta Salad, 36
Bruschetta, Mashed Fava Bean, 77
Brussels sprouts
    about, 39
    Shredded Brussels Sprouts Salad, 41
    Turmeric Riced Brussels Sprouts, 42
Burgers, Portobello, 115

C

Cabbage
    about, 43
    Braised Cabbage, Apples, and White Beans, 44
    Quick Sesame-Soy Red Cabbage Slaw, 45
Cardamom-Maple Roasted Baby Carrots, 47
Carrots
    about, 46
    Cardamom-Maple Roasted Baby Carrots, 47
    Roasted Carrot and Tahini Dressing, 48
    Salt and Vinegar Carrot Crisps, 49
Cashew, and Edamame Salad, Spicy Cucumber, 67
Cauliflower
    about, 50
    Cauliflower Mac 'n' "Cheese," 53
    Spiced Cauliflower, Chickpea, and Raisin Salad, 52
    Turmeric Cauliflower Steaks, 51

Celery
  about, 54
  Celery with Almond Butter and Pomegranate Arils, 55
Celery root
  about, 56
  Garlicky Celery Root and Potato Soup, 57
Chard
  about, 58
  Maple Chard Salad, 60
Cherry Dip, Fresh Corn and, 65
Chickpeas
  Spaghetti Squash with Kale and Chickpeas, 165
  Spiced Cauliflower, Chickpea, and Raisin Salad, 52
  Sweet Potato and Chickpea Curry, 151
Chicories
  about, 61
  Escarole and White Bean Soup, 62
Chimichurri, Homemade, 93
Chips
  Crispy Kale Chips, 99
  Mushroom Chips, 113
  Paprika Baked Potato Chips, 136
  Radish Chips, 140
  Salt and Vinegar Carrot Crisps, 49
Cilantro
  Cilantro-Lime Riced Broccoli, 32
  Homemade Chimichurri, 93
Citrusy Microgreens, 149
Coconut milk
  Coconut Braised Kale, 98
  Coconut Curry Golden Beet Soup, 25
Collards
  about, 97
  Gumbo Z'Herbes, 101

Corn
  about, 63
  Corn Chowder, 64
  Fresh Corn and Cherry Dip, 65
Cranberry and Wild Rice Stuffing, Acorn Squash with, 164
Cucumbers
  about, 66
  Cucumber-Melon Salsa, 68
  Spicy Cucumber, Cashew, and Edamame Salad, 67
Curry
  Coconut Curry Golden Beet Soup, 25
  Okra Curry, 117
  Sweet Potato and Chickpea Curry, 151

D

Dijon mustard
  Maple-Mustard Roasted Turnips, 161
  Snap Pea and Barley Salad with Shallot Dijon Vinaigrette, 128
Dill, Sautéed Green Peas with, 127
Dips
  Fresh Corn and Cherry Dip, 65
  Pureed Turnip and Garlic Dip, 162
Dressing, Roasted Carrot and Tahini, 48

E

Edamame Salad, Spicy Cucumber, Cashew, and, 67
Eggplants
  about, 69
  Eggplant Bacon, 70
  Eggplant Parmesan, 71
  Japanese Eggplant with Thai Basil, 72

Endive
  about, 73
  Braised Endive, 74
Escarole and White Bean Soup, 62

F

Fava beans
  about, 75
  Marinated Fava Beans, 78
  Mashed Fava Bean Bruschetta, 77
Fennel
  about, 79
  Roasted Fennel and Tomatoes over Pasta, 80
Flavorings, 4
Fries
  Baked Jicama Fries with Homemade Chimichurri, 95
  Beet Fries with Garlic Tahini, 27

G

Garlic
  about, 81
  All-Purpose Garlic Marinade, 83
  Beet Fries with Garlic Tahini, 27
  Garlicky Celery Root and Potato Soup, 57
  Pureed Turnip and Garlic Dip, 162
  Roasted Garlic Bulbs, 82
Ginger
  about, 84
  Homemade Candied Ginger, 85
  Rhubarb and Candied Ginger Jam, 142
Gnocchi, Sweet Potato, 154
Gravy, Mushroom and Lentil, 114

Index   175

Green beans
  about, 86
  Blackened Green Beans, 87
  Green Beans and Potatoes, 88
Greens, 97
Grilling, 5
Grocery shopping, 2–3
Gumbo Z'Herbes, 101

H

Herbs
  about, 89
  Cilantro-Lime Riced Broccoli, 32
  DIY Dried Herbs, 92
  Fresh Bell Pepper and Herb Salad, 131
  Frozen Olive Oil and Rosemary Cubes, 91
  Homemade Chimichurri, 93
  Japanese Eggplant with Thai Basil, 72
  Sautéed Green Peas with Dill, 127
  Tarragon Roasted Radishes, 139
  Thyme Roasted Parsnip Coins, 124

J

Jam, Rhubarb and Candied Ginger, 142
Jicama
  about, 94
  Baked Jicama Fries with Homemade Chimichurri, 95
  Jicama-Mango Salsa, 96

K

Kale
  about, 97
  Coconut Braised Kale, 98
  Crispy Kale Chips, 99
  Gumbo Z'Herbes, 101
  Spaghetti Squash with Kale and Chickpeas, 165
Kohlrabi
  about, 102
  Kohlrabi Noodles with Red Sauce and Kidney Beans, 103

L

Leeks
  about, 104
  Roasted Leeks, 105
Lentils
  French Lentil and Shallot Soup, 122
  Mushroom and Lentil Gravy, 114
Lettuce
  about, 107
  Grilled Romaine Lettuce, 110
  Vermicelli Lettuce Wraps, 109
Linguine with Asparagus, 20

M

Mango Salsa, Jicama-, 96
Maple syrup
  Cardamom-Maple Roasted Baby Carrots, 47
  Maple Chard Salad, 60
  Maple-Mustard Roasted Turnips, 161
  Roasted Baby Bok Choy with Spicy Maple Miso, 30
Marinade, All-Purpose Garlic, 83
Melon Salsa, Cucumber-, 68
Microgreens
  about, 148
  Citrusy Microgreens, 149
Miso, Roasted Baby Bok Choy with Spicy Maple, 30
Mushrooms
  about, 111
  Balsamic Roasted Mushrooms, 112
  Mushroom and Lentil Gravy, 114
  Mushroom Chips, 113
  Portobello Burgers, 115
Mustard. *See* Dijon mustard
Mustard greens
  Gumbo Z'Herbes, 101
  Sautéed Mustard Greens, 100

O

Okra
  about, 116
  Okra Curry, 117
Olive oil
  Frozen Olive Oil and Rosemary Cubes, 91
  Olive Oil Purple Potato Salad, 135
Onions
  about, 118
  Avocado Toast with Quick Pickled Red Onions, 23
  Make-Ahead Caramelized Onions, 119
  Quick Pickled Red Onions, 121

P

Pancakes, Scallion, 106
Paprika Baked Potato Chips, 136
Parsnips
  about, 123
  Parsnip and Apple Soup, 125
  Thyme Roasted Parsnip Coins, 124
Pasta and noodles
  Broccolini Pasta Salad, 36
  Cauliflower Mac 'n' "Cheese," 53
  Kohlrabi Noodles with Red Sauce and Kidney Beans, 103

Index

Linguine with Asparagus, 20
Pumpkin Pasta
   Carbonara, 166
Roasted Fennel and
   Tomatoes over Pasta, 80
Sweet Potato Gnocchi, 154
Vermicelli Lettuce
   Wraps, 109
Zucchini Pesto Pasta, 169
Peanut Salad, Shaved
   Rutabaga and, 144
Peanut Sauce, Steamed
   Broccoli with, 33
Peas and peapods
   about, 126
   Asparagus Soup with Peas, 19
   Sautéed Green Peas
      with Dill, 127
   Snap Pea and Barley
      Salad with Shallot Dijon
      Vinaigrette, 128
Peppers, 129. *See also*
   Bell peppers
Pesto Pasta, Zucchini, 169
Pickled Red Onions, Quick, 121
Pine Nut Salad, Shaved
   Asparagus and, 18
Pineapple Avocado Salad, 22
Pizza Crust, Sweet Potato, 153
Pomegranate Arils, Celery with
   Almond Butter and, 55
Posole Verde, 156
Potatoes. *See also*
      Sweet potatoes
   about, 133
   Garlicky Celery Root and
      Potato Soup, 57
   Green Beans and
      Potatoes, 88
   Olive Oil Purple Potato
      Salad, 135
   Paprika Baked Potato
      Chips, 136
   Scalloped Potatoes, 137
Pumpkin Pasta Carbonara, 166

R

Radishes
   about, 138
   Radish Chips, 140
   Tarragon Roasted
      Radishes, 139
Raisin Salad, Spiced Cauliflower,
   Chickpea, and, 52
Rhubarb
   about, 141
   Rhubarb and Candied
      Ginger Jam, 142
Roasting, 5
Romanesco, 50
Rosemary Cubes, Frozen
   Olive Oil and, 91
Rutabagas
   about, 143
   Shaved Rutabaga and
      Peanut Salad, 144

S

Salads
   Broccolini Pasta Salad, 36
   Fresh Bell Pepper and
      Herb Salad, 131
   Maple Chard Salad, 60
   Olive Oil Purple Potato
      Salad, 135
   Pineapple Avocado Salad, 22
   Quick Sesame-Soy Red
      Cabbage Slaw, 45
   Shaved Asparagus and
      Pine Nut Salad, 18
   Shaved Rutabaga and
      Peanut Salad, 144
   Shredded Brussels
      Sprouts Salad, 41
   Snap Pea and Barley
      Salad with Shallot Dijon
      Vinaigrette, 128
   Spiced Cauliflower, Chickpea,
      and Raisin Salad, 52
   Spicy Cucumber, Cashew,
      and Edamame Salad, 67

Salsas
   Arugula Salsa Verde, 15
   Cucumber-Melon
      Salsa, 68
   Jicama-Mango Salsa, 96
   Salt and Vinegar Carrot
      Crisps, 49
Sauces
   Homemade Chimichurri, 93
   Homemade Tomato
      Sauce, 158
   Mushroom and Lentil
      Gravy, 114
Sautéing, 5
Scallions
   about, 104
   Scallion Pancakes, 106
Seasonal shopping, 3
Sesame-Soy Red Cabbage
   Slaw, Quick, 45
Shallots
   about, 118
   French Lentil and
      Shallot Soup, 122
   Snap Pea and Barley
      Salad with Shallot Dijon
      Vinaigrette, 128
Soups
   Asparagus Soup with
      Peas, 19
   Coconut Curry Golden
      Beet Soup, 25
   Corn Chowder, 64
   Escarole and White
      Bean Soup, 62
   French Lentil and
      Shallot Soup, 122
   Garden Tomato Soup, 159
   Garlicky Celery Root and
      Potato Soup, 57
   Parsnip and Apple
      Soup, 125
   Stuffed Pepper Soup, 132
Spaghetti Squash with Kale
   and Chickpeas, 165

Index   **177**

Spinach
   about, 145
   Easy Wilted Spinach, 146
   Spinach and White
      Bean Stir-Fry, 147
Sprouts, 148
Squash. See Summer squash;
   Winter squash; Zucchini
Steaming, 5
Stir-Fry, Spinach and
   White Bean, 147
Stir-frying, 5
Stuffing, Acorn Squash
   with Cranberry and
   Wild Rice, 164
Summer squash, 167
Sweet potatoes
   about, 150
   Sweet Potato and
      Chickpea Curry, 151
   Sweet Potato Gnocchi, 154
   Sweet Potato Pizza Crust, 153

T

Tahini
   Beet Fries with Garlic
      Tahini, 27
   Roasted Carrot and
      Tahini Dressing, 48
Tarragon Roasted Radishes, 139

Teriyaki Tofu and Roasted
   Broccoli, 34
Thai Basil, Japanese
   Eggplant with, 72
Thyme Roasted Parsnip
   Coins, 124
Toast with Quick Pickled Red
   Onions, Avocado, 23
Tofu
   Teriyaki Tofu and Roasted
      Broccoli, 34
   Vermicelli Lettuce
      Wraps, 109
Tomatillos
   about, 155
   Arugula Salsa Verde, 15
   Posole Verde, 156
Tomatoes
   about, 157
   Garden Tomato Soup, 159
   Homemade Tomato
      Sauce, 158
   Roasted Fennel and
      Tomatoes over Pasta, 80
Tools and equipment, 6
Turmeric
   Turmeric Cauliflower
      Steaks, 51
   Turmeric Riced Brussels
      Sprouts, 42

Turnips
   about, 160
   Maple-Mustard Roasted
      Turnips, 161
   Pureed Turnip and
      Garlic Dip, 162

V

Vermicelli Lettuce Wraps, 109
Vinegar Carrot Chips,
   Salt and, 49

W

Wild Rice Stuffing,
   Acorn Squash with
   Cranberry and, 164
Winter squash
   about, 163
   Acorn Squash with Cranberry
      and Wild Rice Stuffing, 164
   Pumpkin Pasta Carbonara, 166
   Spaghetti Squash with Kale
      and Chickpeas, 165

Z

Zucchini
   about, 167
   Zucchini Boats, 170
   Zucchini Pesto Pasta, 169

About the Author

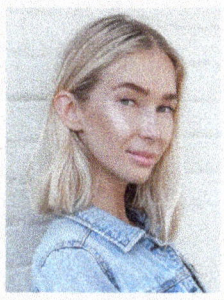 Larissa Olczak is a health and wellness blogger, recipe developer, and author. Her popular first book, *Easy Vegetable Meals*, can be found on Amazon and all major bookstores. She started a company called I Am Well by Larissa where she helps clients become more conscious of their health by providing education on holistic wellness, herbs, nutrition, and lifestyle. She graduated from California State University, Northridge, with a communications degree and continued to become a Nutritional Therapy Practitioner at the Nutritional Therapy Association.

www.ingramcontent.com/pod-product-compliance
Lightning Source LLC
Chambersburg PA
CBHW050259090426
42735CB00024B/3491